Mystic Awakening of an American Physician

by

Linda Hostalek, D.O.

Mystic Awakening of an AmericanPhysician

Mystic Awakening of an AmericanPhysician
Linda Hostalek, D.O.

Mystic Awakening of an AmericanPhysician

ii

Mystic Awakening of an AmericanPhysician
Linda Hostalek, D.O.

Acknowledgements

There are so many people to whom I owe thanks on
this work of my heart, I love you all and appreciate
each of you. First of all, thank you to the Creator, for
giving me the experiences and the courage to bare
my soul for all to see, and to Pachamama for all my
needs met. Thank you to Richard, for bringing these
experiences into my life. Thank you to Jose Luis, for
many healings, teachings, prayers and friendship
during this profound journey. To Bill, my 'energy dad,'
for his love and support in bringing this creation to
fruition, and to my mom and dad, for their support
throughout my life, and the many blessings of
unconditional love they have shown me. To my four
children: Jim, Michael, Derek and David, who have
shown me how to love beyond time. To Betsy, Joyce,

Mystic Awakening of an AmericanPhysician

and Brian, for numerous hours of editing and encouragement, and to Michael for bringing the cover design to fruition. To the land, sea and sky for giving me life and a sense of purpose, and to you, dear reader, for buying this book and holding the option to transform your life and those around you. Thank you.

Mystic Awakening of an AmericanPhysician
Linda Hostalek, D.O.

Prologue

This is the story of a mystic awakened. Based on a
true story, this book is designed to take the reader on
a journey through the eyes of the spiritual seeker,
opening up in response to revelations in her spirit.
Set during my time in medical school, trying to make
sense of all that life entails, I have done my best to
capture the sense of awakening and awe that inspired
this creation. In some instances, names or other
information may have been slightly changed for
artistic license. My prayer is that you will feel the
illumination of your own spirit as you read these
pages, and that the mystic inside you will awaken, or
re-awaken, and make itself known.

Mystic Awakening of an AmericanPhysician

Chapter 1

Healing is More Than Just the Body

It was a relatively ordinary day. I stopped by the coffee shop on my way home from school to study, and had some chai tea. As a single mom with four boys at home I often stopped by after school before I went home to my 'second shift.' I did a little studying, and picked up a couple of the local free magazines that were in the display bin by the door. I shoved them in my backpack, and set out the door for home.

The kids were home, so we did our normal stuff, eat, homework, talk/play and then bed. Once they were asleep, I went to my room, and opened my backpack. I took out the text I was studying, as I often studied in bed before I went to sleep.

The magazines slipped out onto the floor, I was too tired to care. I took a shower and got ready for bed.

Mystic Awakening of an AmericanPhysician

As I settled in, and was ready to pick up my book and study, I noticed the picture on the back of the magazine on the floor. Although an ordinary picture, my soul was mesmerized. It was a picture of a man on a horse, in the mountains. He was a doctor who did some mission work in the Andes with Q'ero people, the descendants of the Inka. He was also a shaman, and was giving a lecture at the end of the week in a nearby bookstore called Blue Feather. I knew deep in my heart that this was going to change my life. I didn't know how, or how radically, but I just had to go check this out. I had learned by then to trust my instincts when they were that clear.

I was in medical school at the time, deciding to utilize my talents for healing. I had always been a bit of a mystic, having the ability to sense and see energy fields. When I was about six years old, I remember seeing a beautiful glow of colors around this loving spirit of a woman. She told me that I was from the Pleides because of my blond hair and blue eyes, and my ability to see auras. I didn't know at the time what an 'aura' was, but I was in the pure flow of a child,

and the blues, greens, and purply-pink of her energy
field amazed me.

Through different energetic traditions, such as Reiki,
QiGong, and Kriya yoga, I learned about the chakra
system and the centers, or tiens, of energetic
vortexes in the human body. Chakras are condensed
electromagnetic fields on the body that interact with
the world, the being and the many layers of the
human energetic system, including the physical body,
the emotional body, the astral body, and the like.
During that time, I studied Reiki, an ancient Japanese
healing art and became a master-teacher of that
ancient healing discipline. I enjoyed it very much
because energy fields were used to heal people in
that ancient discipline of laying on of hands.

In medical school, I was vastly immersed in the field
of cranial osteopathy, another very energetic
discipline, working with the field through the cranial
rhythm, the basic rhythm of the life force. There is an
inherent rhythm of life, called the cranial rhythm,
distinct from the other rhythms of life such as pulse
and respirations. One had to have 'hands' to palpate

this very subtle energetic rhythm, but once one learned to read the language of the body, it would tell you everything. It was through the Cranial Academy that I learned how to use Vogel crystals, specialized quartz crystals programmed with love and healing, to balance energetic fields.

Crystals in particular, and rocks in general had always appealed to me, so I studied through Rumi Da, an apprentice of Marcel Vogel himself, who carried on his work after his death. I had a very special Vogel crystal that I called 'Pinky.' Another aspect of the field was the Osteopathic percussion hammer, an advanced form of cranial made popular by the famous Dr. Robert Fulford, a cranial osteopath who paved the way for forward thinking through the Cranial Academy. The vibrating percussive head resonates with the vibrational signature of the human body, enabling great healings to occur under the right conditions.

Impressions of medical states had begun to be impressed into me, and taught me that healing involves much more than just the body. There is a transcendent force that leads to a balance of all the

Mystic Awakening of an AmericanPhysician
Linda Hostalek, D.O.

different layers of being involved in the healing process. The truths began to coalesce for me prior to medical school. I had studied very intently in both school and in the mystery schools during my time prior to and during medical school, reading every book on healing, including shamanism, that I could.

Having had a bout with cancer, and facing possible death, combined with my inherent abilities, the veil became increasingly thin. As angels held me in the hospital, I remember hearing "this is so you will be a better doctor." I was not yet in medical school, but I intuitively knew that there was more at work in my healing from this dis-ease than just the surgery, radiation, and chemo. As I learned more about energy my fields became clearer, and I began to see similar emotional patterns in people with certain clusters of illnesses. I wanted to learn how to heal those patterns, not just in my life, but in others as well. Intuitively I understood that healing is more than just the body, but needed to be integrated on all levels, and I wanted to learn more.

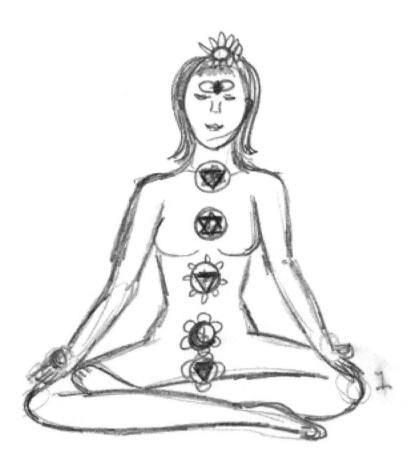

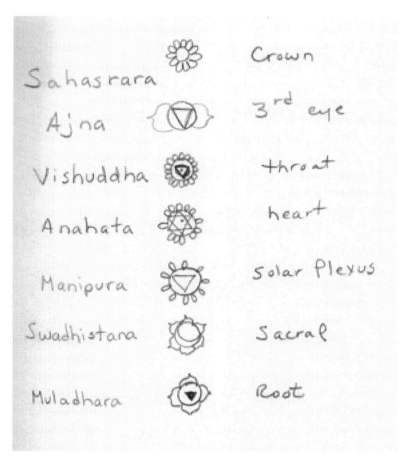

Sahasrara		Crown
Ajna		3rd eye
Vishuddha		throat
Anahata		heart
Manipura		solar plexus
Swadhistana		Sacral
Muladhara		Root

****first chakra*****

My first clinical rotation was surgery, and as I sat there waiting for my supervising doctor to arrive, I noticed a man walking across the room. His name was Henry and I noticed an energy in him that jumped to me as

Mystic Awakening of an AmericanPhysician

'hemorrhoids' from an ethereal source. I thought that was interesting, and it was kinda funny and tickled inside. I had been able to ascertain emotions from people in the past, but this was the first time spirit had talked to me so forcefully about a physical condition.

I watched the particular way Henry walked, with an uptightness that led to a very narrow pelvic movement. I also noticed that his root chakra was closed, as well as a density in his luminous body. As I sat there, observing Henry, the supervising doctor, Dr. Jones, arrived and we began to see patients. Henry was the first one we saw. He was rather short at 5'4', mid thirties with a stocky build, a mop of dark, somewhat messy hair and dark suspicious eyes. He didn't want to be here, and gave off the impression of a nearly paranoid personality. He was a computer engineer, and had an air of superiority about him, but kept looking around as if someone was out to get him. He had had this pain before, and he kept it to himself, and now it was too overwhelming. He went to see his primary doctor and he was given a creme, but it didn't do the job. His family physician sent him over to get it looked at. He was worried this would cost a lot. He had taken a day off work, and his "boss didn't like" him anyway. In fact, the more he talked, he felt like no one liked him, especially women. He looked at me suspiciously, "you don't know what it's like to be me", he said, "you've got it made being an attractive woman. You get to get your meals paid for and go on vacation, and promotions all because of your nice 'smile', that never happens to us guys".

Dr. Jones interrupted him, "Let's see what we have here" he said.

When Henry dropped his pants and bent over, two big, fat hemorrhoids pulsated slowly, like red, ugly worms. "How long is this gonna take, doc, I can't miss anymore work, can you give me a creme like my other doctor did before, only stronger?".
"No, Henry, those are going to need surgery to remove, I'll have the nurse come in and get you the details," Dr. Jones said.

When we left the room, Dr. Jones told me his other doctor had tried to get him to take care of his bowel habits, not strain, and eat more fiber, but when they (hemorrhoids) aren't taken care of while they are small, they grow in to the monsters emerging from this poor guy's butt. I realized that Henry had been dealing with problems related to his base chakra, he felt inferior, didn't trust people and felt like a victim, especially now that his body had 'betrayed' him. I realized that the energetic fields can 'talk' if we only listen. I was ready to listen, and I began to learn a lot.

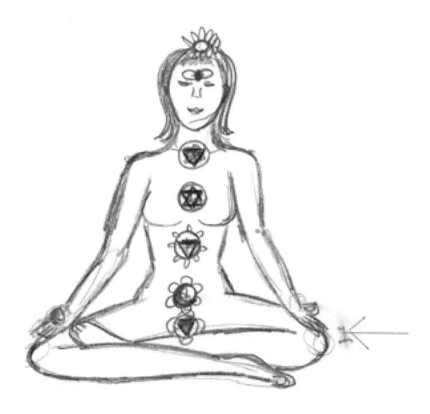

Mystic Awakening of an AmericanPhysician
Linda Hostalek, D.O.

****second chakra****

My next rotation was gynecology, the studies of women's health. Mostly a lot of pap smears and pelvic exams, but here I began to see how energetically a woman's belief in her sexuality affected her sexual health. I would find this to be true also with men, but there were no men on this rotation. Some of the women were very happy in their relationship with their partner, and their life. Only rarely was there ever a 'problem' with these women, mostly just yearly check-ups.

I began to notice a pattern with these women's relationship to themselves, as well as their partners, to their physical health. I would see that some of these women really didn't like the relationship they were in. They would give their power away, and kinda just die inside. One girl, I'll call Tanesha, was a 19 year old high school dropout with a three year old child, a part time job as a cashier at a convenience store, and had a strained relationship with the baby's father, to whom she was not married to. She was living with her mom, and some siblings, trying to get by. She felt stuck "What am I supposed to do?" she said.

"What do you mean?" I asked.

"I have a baby to take care of, my mom needs my help, and that son-of-a-bitch can't make up his mind between me and that bitch Nancy."
"You have a lot on your plate", I said.

"Yeah. I love him, so I stay with him, but sometimes I just wish I could just escape. I don't do no drugs anymore, not since I've been pregnant, and my baby girl is going on three this September".

She had gotten herpes, and didn't know if it was from her baby's father, or from some other guy she had recently had casual sex with for a few months now after her 'baby-daddy' started sleeping again with her one-time friend. Energetically her pelvis looked like a black hole, so dense, so much pain, yet seething with emotional distrust. I asked her, "Do you have any hobbies? What do you do for fun?"

Mystic Awakening of an AmericanPhysician
Linda Hostalek, D.O.

"I used to sing at my church, and dance, I don't do that anymore, and haven't in a while. I just don't feel like singing anymore". We finished our visit, and I tried to encourage her to start singing again. I never saw her again after that.

There were a few women there with AIDS, one was a drug addict, who made her living as a stripper. She was disgusted with herself and how she was living her life. To her men were an ends to their means, usually money or drugs. She appeared to feel so guilty and ashamed. "My mother doesn't even know I'm sick," she said, "wouldn't matter, all she cares about is booze anyway."

"What about your father?" I asked.

I knew I touched on hurtful subject when she retorted, "My dad used to call me a princess, then it was don't tell mommy, now its don't even talk to me, you're a slut-- but I wasn't a slut when He was the one fucking me, yeah, I'm some princess all right!"

Mystic Awakening of an AmericanPhysician

"When was the last time you've seen either of them?"

"I haven't seen either one in years, probably five years or so for my dad, and he can rot in hell for all I care!"

All I could see was the hate and guilt literally eating her up. She could not forgive. The pain in her field could fill a room. She masked it the only way she knew how, with drugs to dull the pain and the memories. Her dark cloud over her pelvis had stretched to include her entire dense, dark luminous field. Unable to forgive, the resentment she felt turned on herself to cause her to die; first inside, and now in this reality, causing her immune system to turn on herself. I could only pray she could find a way to forgive those that had hurt her, and herself as well.

Another woman, I'll call her "Evelyn", was recovering from cervical cancer. She was a tall, thin, lithe woman, with thin, blond hair, cut into a short bob, age 52. She was dressed nice, but casual, and worked as a graphic artist in the city for a very prominent company. She was recently divorced, and now seeing someone new, and was rather nervous about having sex with a new partner. Her now ex-husband had cheated on her with a younger woman, and the divorce occurred after that. She was devastated, as she had just learned of her cancer, and had her procedures, and was looking forward to life after that scare with the man she married and planned a life with.

After that came the revelation of the affair. Her husband left, and she was devastated. More than able to provide for herself financially, she found herself in a new place of vulnerability. She was unable to concentrate on her work, and lost a few key clients during this time. She had already had considerable time off already dealing with her illness, and now she was having to remake her life while trying to stay focused enough to be productive at work.

"How did you get through all that?" I asked.

She said to me, "I just had to pull myself up by my bootstraps, and just carry on during the day, but when

Mystic Awakening of an AmericanPhysician

I came home to the huge, empty house, all I wanted to do at first was cry."

"That sounds very painful, but brave." I said. "What did you do next?"

"I got hurt, then angry." she said. "I felt old, ugly, and unlovable, I even contemplated suicide for a short while, really just a moment, but then I thought there is no way I am going to give that son of a bitch the satisfaction of that. I decided I had to make my life over, and to learn from this experience. I was worth it. I have 2 grown children, a son in college, and a daughter in residency, and I said it's my time now."

"So what do you do with your time now?".

"I read books and watched some tapes on yoga, and decided to learn how to do that. Now I do my practice everyday, almost, and I've even been to a yoga retreat! I can do my work again, because I am grateful for learning what was important to me, and who was important to me. Things didn't work out with my ex and his new girlfriend, and now he's realized he made a mistake, and is trying to make things up to me, but I'm not sure that's what I want."

"So what do you want?" I asked.

"To be happy. I met a man a few months ago, and I'm scared, but I don't want to be; so I'm going to try to live life how I want, not what other's expectations of me are. I just want to be sure I'm all okay 'down there' before I begin to take this new relationship to the next level".

"Wow!", I thought, this lady has been through so much, and here she is, in her mid-fifties having the time of her life discovering who she really is. Although her physical condition had left her a bit scarred, there was no disease, and from a medical point of view she was ready for sex. From an energetic point of view, she was too, a vibrant, orange glow was evident in her pelvis, and I'm sure she made the right decisions for her. These three different women showed me that how you feel about yourself, irrespective of what another thinks of you, especially

from a sexual or creative stance, will greatly influence
your health.

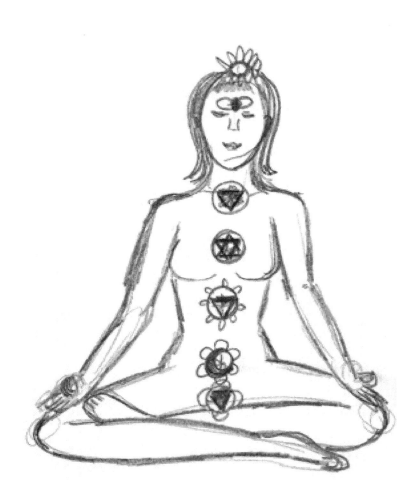

Mystic Awakening of an AmericanPhysician
Linda Hostalek, D.O.

****third chakra****

The following rotation was internal medicine, basically taking care of people with multiple types of acute illnesses, including those in intensive care. One lady came in with abdominal pain, digestive issues, and a moderate yellowing of her skin. She had some problems with her liver and pancreas, and had jaundice, a yellowing of the skin, which on her progressed to a very strange, almost florescent yellow-orange. She looked like a pumpkin. The pumpkin lady's name was Gladys, and she was a tough acting, 62 year old caucasian female somewhat plump with wild gray hair and piercing green eyes, made even more intense by the whites of her eyes being yellow. Widowed, and with no family around, she arrived in the ER by a caring neighbor who was concerned because she just didn't 'look right.' Full of anger and spite, she cussed like a sailor and let you know what was wrong-- and everything was, the food, the temperature, the way the nurses treated her. She didn't want to be here, and she let everyone know it.

Mystic Awakening of an AmericanPhysician

She was assigned to me, and I would make my
rounds daily, and eventually she became somewhat
friendly with me (meaning she didn't curse at me, very
much anyway, when I walked in to her room!). I came
to know that she had been a seamstress for over 50
years, then her eyesight became so bad she could no
longer do her job. Her husband did carpentry work,
but died of a heart attack about 5 years ago. Her
children lived on opposite coasts and didn't visit
much. She used to play bridge with her friends, but
now her eyes were so bad she couldn't see the cards.
She had a fire inside of her, but also anger,
resentment and guilt. A dark, heavy energy fell over
her solar plexus, as well as her heart.

This lady had been through a lot. She was is in the
hospital for over a month, and needed a procedure on
her pancreas. When her family heard of her
hospitalization, her children made arrangement to
come visit her, I noticed her gradually 'softening.' The
next morning when I went in to do my daily rounds on
her, she was crying. "Gladys?" I asked, "What's
wrong?"

Mystic Awakening of an American Physician
Linda Hostalek, D.O.

"I don't want to talk now," she barked, "Leave me alone!" I thought of perhaps doing that, but sensed she needed to 'let it out', so I came to her bed and sat down, and then she just sobbed and sobbed and sobbed. "I've been such a bad person, I was a bad wife, I was a bad mother, I'm useless, and I can't hardly even see anymore!"

This was quite a change from the crotchety old lady I'd grown accustomed to. The hard shell around the marshmallow was melting.

"Now why would you say that?" I asked, secretly happy she was opening up, even if it meant some tears needed to be shed.

"What if I die and never got to tell the people I love that I love them?" she sobbed. "I don't know how to do that. I mean I think they know, but I just don't know how to tell them. And what if they don't love me back?"

"Sometimes all you can do is say how you feel and go from there. Maybe they need you to say it first?"

"I suppose," she said, wiping the tears from her face, as a small smile tried to appear. "They did come all the way here to see me, even when I haven't been all that nice to them lately."

"You can always start today," I said, as I finished my daily exam. It was a pleasure to watch her and her family begin to reconnect.

We talked a little bit about letting go of old hurts, and living for today, and making relationships count, as no one was sure if she would live through this. She was the most brightly colored pigmented color of a human I have ever seen; to say she was florescent would be an understatement! After this encounter, she was happier, and began talking to her kids. They remarked they were worried about their mom, and they too, began to melt as they expressed their love for their mom from their heart. She began to lose some of her bright yellow color, and that dark glob of energy over her third chakra or solar plexus (also called the manipura chakra).

Mystic Awakening of an AmericanPhysician
Linda Hostalek, D.O.

This lady, who we pretty much expected to die, recovered in her body, mind and soul, at least enough to leave the hospital. She no longer appeared to feel anger at herself or guilt over her past. She had rekindled the relationship with her family and now actually smiled! It was a happy day when she was released. I don't know what happened to her after that, but I was thrilled to witness the recovery of her soul, which led to the recovery of her physical body. Now when I think of Gladys, I think of the wonderful power of love and forgiveness on healing. She still reminds me of a luminous light bulb, although this time its in her heart instead of her skin.

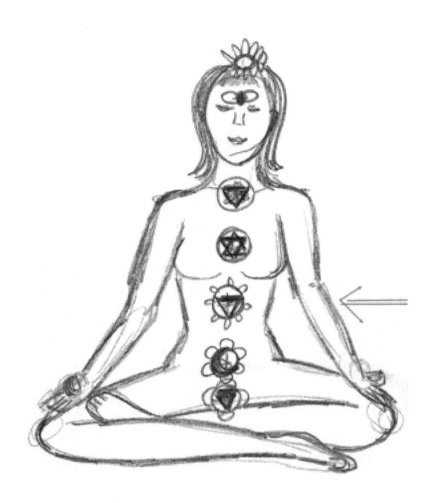

Mystic Awakening of an AmericanPhysician
Linda Hostalek, D.O.

****fourth chakra****

Another encounter showed me another aspect of the emotional aspect of health and healing. A man named Gene, late 50's, divorced, nonsmoker, weight appropriate business owner, came in with a heart attack. He was about 5'11", well dressed, handsome man with greying salt and pepper hair, and strong features.

Chest pain was a pretty common condition in the hospital. If the ER released them to our care we usually would just watch them overnight and if all was well, let them go the next day. Gene had pain that just would not go away, so he was scheduled for a heart cath, a procedure to see if there is blockage. There was not. His cardiac enzymes were normal, but he had this feeling of 'impending doom,' like he was going to die. "I don't know what's wrong with me, doc, I just don't feel right, I can't breathe, my chest hurts, like there's a gorilla there that won't leave me alone".

Mystic Awakening of an AmericanPhysician

It turns out this was the monthly anniversary of his divorce 5 years ago, and his mothers death 3 years ago. He was worried about his kids, they were in college, and was having a bit of a financial struggle with the dealership, and trying to keep it all together.

"I've always been an over-achiever, but what has it gotten me? My wife left me, said I didn't spend enough 'quality time' with her", he said snidely, "I work my ass off to give my kids everything I didn't have, and they get mad because the car I gave him was the wrong kind, I mean, come on, doc, what's a guy to do? Then my mom had been sick, dad died about 5 years prior, and I mean, she's my mom, I had to take care of her, she sacrificed so I could go to college and get a good job, I mean, the woman was a saint, and probably the only one who ever really loved me."
A tear rolled from his eye. It was five years to the day that his mother had died. He wasn't at the bedside when it happened, he was at work. He hadn't yet forgiven himself. He apologized for crying, "I'm sorry, doc, I don't usually do this."

Mystic Awakening of an AmericanPhysician
Linda Hostalek, D.O.

"It's okay," I said. "Heartfelt tears are beautiful displays of emotions, and very cleansing." Realizing that he probably didn't take the time to feel his emotions very often, I said "It's important to acknowledge your feelings." The beauty of his tears nearly made me cry too. This man had given himself away to everyone else, and didn't know how to love himself. He worked to provide, that was his way of showing love to those he cared about.

"Stress, especially continuous emotional stress, makes certain chemicals in your body, like cortisol and clotting factors that can lead to very physical issues in your heart, such as those that can lead to a heart attack. Emotional peace and happiness can have the opposite effect." I put my hand on his as I continued, "Sometimes we just need to forgive ourselves and others too to free up that emotional space in our heart. We can only do the best we can under the conditions that we are in presently."

"I never thought of it that way before. Just do the best you can," he said, as he sighed with a smile. "I can do that."

Mystic Awakening of an AmericanPhysician

As we spoke, the empty, dark space in his chest began to fill up with life again. We talked more about the relationship between the physical heart and the emotional one. He still loved his ex-wife, and wanted his family whole. I don't know if he ever achieved that, but from that brief encounter, the healing that happened had appeared to change him. He was no longer anxious, and could see how all these emotional aspects had affected him.

For me, I was mesmerized watching the energy fill back in as he made his connections between the emotional patterns. Love is the most healing vibration. As I watched this man begin to forgive and love himself, the healing began. If you are out there Gene, I hope you are happy and well, and have found the peace you were looking for.

Mystic Awakening of an AmericanPhysician
Linda Hostalek, D.O.

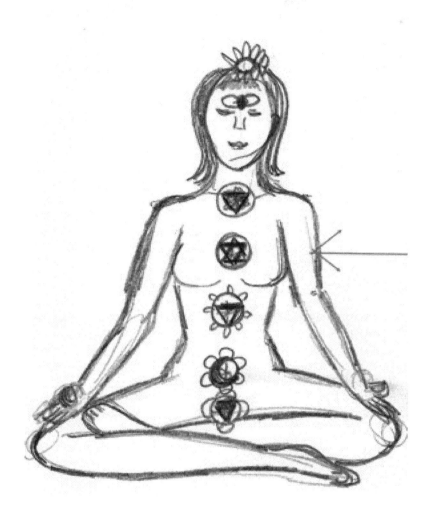

Mystic Awakening of an AmericanPhysician

****fifth chakra****

Another remarkable patient was a lady named Pattie.
Pattie was a sweet, soft spoken woman, with a short,
chubby body and bright red hair. She was in to see
the doctor about this lump in her throat that wouldn't
go away. It had slowly grown larger over the previous
year. She had gained about 50 pounds, which was
very distressing to her, especially because she only
had a 5'2" frame. This happened shorty after the birth
of her second child. She had a difficult pregnancy,
and had not felt well since. Her child, a little girl
named Iris, was now two years old.

Pattie was married to Fred, an insurance salesman,
and a loud, boisterous, controlling character. He
brought her in, and answered most of the questions
for her.

He said "My wife's not been right since the birth of our
daughter, you gotta help her, she don't do anything
anymore, the house is always a mess, and she don't
want to get with me, if you know what I mean...."

Mystic Awakening of an AmericanPhysician
Linda Hostalek, D.O.

We did some minor testing and discovered her thyroid was enlarged. No cancer appeared to be there, but it needed to get resolved. We gave her some thyroid medicine, and saw her back in a couple of weeks.

She was felling better, a bit more energetic, but now I could see this energetic 'thrust' wanting to come out of her throat. At the time it confused me a little, since she was so much better physically.

Fred had to use the restroom, so it gave us a few minutes alone, when she said "I just don't know what to do, I can't stand the way he talks to me, yet I don't know what to do. He doesn't listen to me, its like I can't have my own opinions," her face red with frustration, contrasted against her red hair,then she let out a big sigh, "huh!" she puffed.

Now it made sense, she may be physically better, but needed to address the spiritual and emotional issues that caused the imbalance in the first place. "We disagree on how to raise the children", she went on, "he thinks I'm his slave, and God forbid If I don't have dinner ready on time!"

"Have you talked to him about how you feel?" I asked.

"No", she said. "Wouldn't do any good anyway, he doesn't listen to me."

I suggested to her to find her 'voice.' "Sometimes just saying it makes it more real", I said to her, and encouraged her to find her truth.

She said "I'll try to, I just can't take this anymore."

I knew that would be a difficult pattern for her to break, but I hope that as she found her truth she could find her voice, and bring the energy back to her throat in so doing that. But, due to the nature of my training, I didn't get to see what happened to her, as I had to moved on to another rotation.

Mystic Awakening of an AmericanPhysician
Linda Hostalek, D.O.

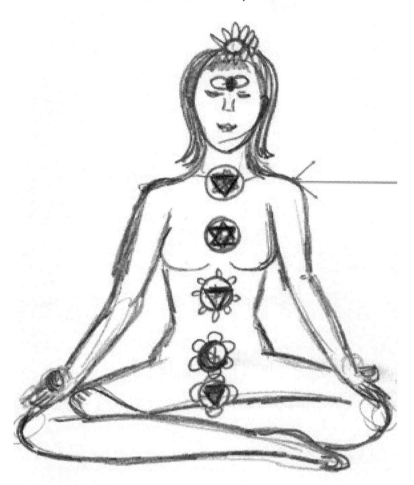

Mystic Awakening of an AmericanPhysician

****sixth chakra****

On the intensive care unit, I was assigned to a
handsome, tall, blond man in his mid-fifties, named
Brian who was admitted the night before with a
stroke. He was a successful businessman, on top of
the world, it would of seem. He had been at a party,
when he began 'not acting right', slurring speech, and
half of his body stopped working.   He was brought in
to the local ER, and was now in the intensive care
unit, and I was assigned to take care of him.

His wife came in, and took charge right away. "I want
the top specialist, the top neurosurgeon taking care of
him!" she demanded. A seasoned professional, she
documented every single thing she witnessed;
people's attitudes, what they brought for him, or
didn't, how often the doctors and nurses would come
in, etc. She wrote down everything I said to her. She
loved her husband very much.

Her name was Jeanie, and was a bright, professional
woman, with warm brown eyes, and long blond hair.
She was a social worker, and was no stranger to the

34

hospital environment. She knew that sometimes you have to be demanding to get what you want. She was by his side daily, and often spent the night. His stroke was the hemorrhagic, or bleeding, type of stroke, and he had lost a significant amount of brain the night before. From here on was the hard part.

The neurosurgeon took him to surgery, and I was allowed the privilege to assist. I was fascinated as I watched the brain pulsate with life, it's own life, almost independent of the body. I was allowed to touch the brain and the spinal cord that was exposed, and it was one of the most special moments of being-ness, of touching creation itself. The pulsations of the brain are not the same as the blood. I had learned this in the Cranial Academy a few years before, but this was on a whole different experiential level of amazing.

My third eye grew that day, teaching me how the brain's intelligence teaches the body and the spirit, and again, how they work together to form a whole. The surgery went well, he now had a shunt to drain off excess fluid, and I rounded on him daily, and kept his wife updated as well. I watched as he opened up consciously, talking was difficult, almost impossible at first, but he progressed to full words then to sentences.

He sat upright and had physical and occupational therapy daily. His wife made sure they brought him all the right stuff, and she arranged the rehab place after his stay. You could see the connection between them, and the energy of their ties were beautiful. That was love. I felt connected to them on a spiritual level. They taught me so much. Again, love really does conquer all.

I ran into her at a professional gathering several years later, and Brian has made an almost total recovery, with only some mild memory gaps and a slight limp. He made some major lifestyle changes as well. My third eye opened up even more with the joy of the collective being, that this soul was affected by the love of another, hers, with his, and a little of mine and other's too. We all received a special blessing that went beyond the physical challenge of getting through the physical illness. A spiritual bond was formed, and I am forever grateful.

Mystic Awakening of an AmericanPhysician
Linda Hostalek, D.O.

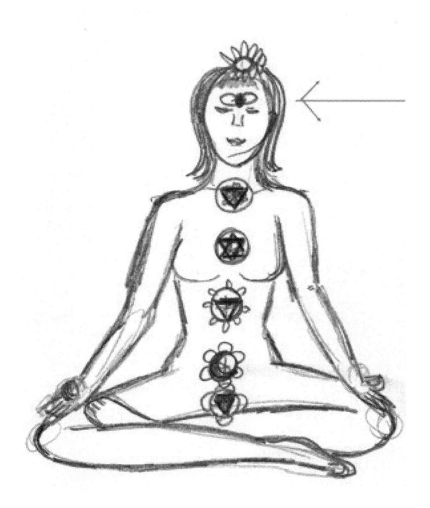

Mystic Awakening of an AmericanPhysician

****seventh chakra****

On another occasion, I rotated with a psychiatrist named Dr. Oppenheimer, which bent my brain in all kinds of knots. Dr. 'O', as he preferred to be called, had the look of a plump, stocky English gentlemen, with brown,slightly gray hair, and a handlebar mustache, which he waxed and twirled to perfection. Well dressed and well spoken, he was known to be a fair and just man and was asked to judge inmates as competent to stand trial, something not too many psychiatrists do routinely.

Depression, anxiety, schizophrenia, trauma, abuse--self or from a perpetrator all took a toll on the brain, as well as the psyche. I noticed certain patterns with different diagnosis, sexual trauma, PTSD, fibromyalgia; basically the body was a diagnostic blueprint of what the soul had witnessed, and how it handled the incidents.

One day I had to go to a prison for the criminally insane for an inmate assessment, this man had

committed a murder by bludgeoning to death another
man, a gang member of a rival gang, with a
sledgehammer. Dr. O had prepped me for this
experience, told me how to act, dress, look, or rather
not look, etc. It was very scary, but a very rare
opportunity for a medical student. We pulled up to the
guard house and our ID's were checked. We drove to
a small building in the back. Images of old school
buildings or of military barracks with a sadistic twist
entered my mind. Armed guards met us outside and
escorted us in.   As we walked through multiple locked
doors, with armed guards all around, I felt relatively
safe. There wasn't any place we went without guards.

Another door, this one a large, heavy, metal door with
multiple locks, opened, and the feeling of safety
lessened greatly. The guards heaved the huge metal
door out of the way and we stepped through.
Although small by prison standards, the hallway I
walked through next was disturbing.

The energy darkened considerably as we walked
through that door. The hallway leading to interview
room was lined with rows of prison cells lining the one

side of the room as we walked by to the next location where we were to meet our patient. I was hit with the locker room like odor of sweat, and blood, pungent in a subtle way, the pheromones releasing fight or flight like tension enhancing molecules inside me. I began to feel very uncomfortable and rather scared, although I dare not show it. I had taken care to make sure I was very professionally dressed, and kept my eyes low as we walked by the cells and the men in them. Dingy grey metal bars, with cement cells, lined the walls, the essence of animalism penetrated every pore.

Male inmates (I saw no females), stared at me, right through me. Their arms reached out through the bars as if trying to grab me. Some yelled "hey blondie", some hooted, some howled, some just looked right through me with dead eyes. I guess it had been a while since any of them had seen an outside person, especially a female.

Dr. O and I were led to a small cell-like room. It was made of cement blocks, painted in what appeared to at one time be white, but was now a sickening yellowing color. This room, too, had the big, steel door and multiple locks. There was a sturdy wooden table with four wooden chairs, much like you would see in any other government institution of the 50's or so.

Two prison guards held our patient, Markus. He was wearing a black and white striped jumpsuit, neatly shaved, with short dark hair and multiple tattoos. He was 6'2, and approximately 250 pounds of pure muscle. He had gang style tattoos on his arms, neck and hands, dark, scarred skin, and eyes that were black and deep, yet not quite there, like his soul was in there somewhere, but had not come out in a very long time. He was in there for murder, he had hacked someone apart over a dispute.

The prison guards led him into the room, unshackled him from both his leg and wrist chains, turned around, and walked out the steel door, and closed it!!! It was just Markus, Dr. O and me! I looked over at Dr. O and he gave me one of those looks that meant, calm down, you will be okay, so I lowered my self into my chair, and listened to my senses and listened to the conversation between the prisoner, our patient, Markus and Dr. O. As Markus spoke to Dr. O, he had a level of humility that betrayed his outer body language. I learned he had suffered great trauma at the hands of parents, clergy, and gang members, and felt he had no recourse other than to give back what he had gotten. One day someone transgressed his territory, and after a warning, it happened again, he dismembered the man. No trace of remorse, it was just a matter of fact. I felt sick inside.

Dr. O asked "Do you hear voices that tell you what to do?"

"No," Markus said, emotionless.

"Do you ever feel like killing yourself or someone else?".

"No."

"Do you feel bad about what you did?"

Mystic Awakening of an AmericanPhysician
Linda Hostalek, D.O.

"No," he said, with a trace of emotion now showing through. "The dude had it coming, I warned him, he should of listened, thats the rule of the streets."
In his mind, what he did was not wrong, just the price that had to be paid.

There were other questions about health, family history, etc, the usual stuff, but I couldn't draw myself away from the energy field of this man. It was very strong, and very tough, and he had overcome a lot. Although his crime was heinous to me, he seemed more like it was just a business transaction to him, although the lack of depth of his energy field indicated to me of an inability to love. His crown chakra cut off, as well as his third eye was dim.

Tragic, numbing, and sad, this person would now spend the rest of his life in prison, where he actually felt safe and secure, in the world he created with his own belief system.

After what seemed like hours, but was in reality about 15 minutes, the steel doors were opened, the guards appeared, re-shackled his ankles and wrists, and walked him out of the door. Dr. O and I stayed in there until he was back in his cell. He could see I was a bit disturbed, and asked me if I was okay.

"I'm okay," I said, and I was; although another chapter in how people use their energy to create their own reality was now written in my soul.

This experience pushed me into accessing my own belief system, and trying to make sense of all this. Eventually I would come to see that we all have choices to make, to be free or not, to harm or not, and to either come to terms with our dysfunctions and learn from them and grow, or continue down the spiral that leads to illness, institutions and spiritual or literal death. I felt a bit shaken from this experience, but it also allowed me to re-evaluate instances in my life that were painful that I had to forgive and let go of. I was also very surprised how much the energy of the prison affected me. It was not a happy place, I found it very, very sad.

Once I was out of there and felt safe again, I was very happy to go back to the normal psyche ward after that and deal with suicide attempts, substance abuse, and

Mystic Awakening of an AmericanPhysician
Linda Hostalek, D.O.

depression. It made me try even harder to help those patients because it was made very clear to me that the one of the possible next step in the evolution of psychiatric illness was to end up like Markus, or one of the other ones moaning, crying, and waiting on death row to die, while they were already dead inside. My prayer is that all the crown chakras would open and become functional and clear, waiting for spiritual guidance to manifest in all healing, helping humanity struggling with such weighty issues.

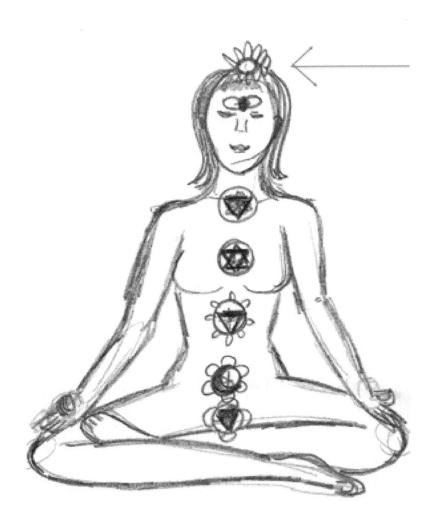

Mystic Awakening of an AmericanPhysician
Linda Hostalek, D.O.

The next several rotations would hone my medical intuitive skill even more. Cancer, pancreatitis, infected gall bladders, appendixes and sinuses each had their own signature, as did depression and schizophrenia. I found the hospitals to be very depressing places, and I started a journal to remember just one thing I was grateful for each day. Having had a personal encounter with cancer, and all the trimmings with it, surgery, radiation, chemo, severe immunosuppression, being in this atmosphere brought out my repressed fears and inner joys. My life was about healing, and first and foremost, that meant healing myself. Journaling an episode of gratitude daily kept me sane and focused, learning that sometimes the slightest little things can bring profound joy, like a baby's cry, or a diabetic's hairy toes (means blood is getting to the toes). Energy is everywhere, in everyone and everything. I was blessed to be able to get an energetic education from spirit during my time there. I was shown how a person's energetic state affects his or her health. Truly the mind, body and spirit are all connected.

Mystic Awakening of an AmericanPhysician

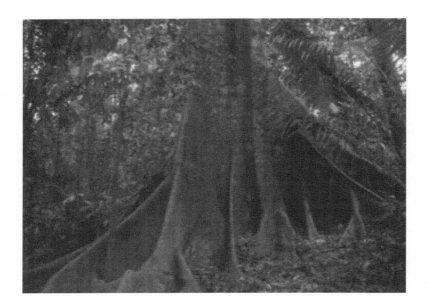

Chapter 2

Beginnings

Always a mystic, I could always see and feel energy, I
thought everyone could the way I did. Being
empathic, I could feel other's pain - which led to a
desire to help them.   I had no idea at the time how
much that helped me to help myself, and learn about
the multiple layers of healing. I found I created
situations to help my personal growth, that at the time
seemed anything but; abuse, trauma, drama, illness,
etc., my life could be a lifetime* movie. Each
archetype I passed through before, during, and after
medical school has taught me a different lesson, but
that is not the focus of this work. What I do want to

emphasize is how I got through all that with the help of spirit, and the many different ways spirit prepared me for this next shift in my life.

During the time when my children were small, we lived in a beautiful home in the country. Situated on 7 acres, the land had a spring, a small creek, woods, fields, and all sorts of wildlife. The plants and animals became my teachers. I would watch as seeds planted were nourished with the love of the earth, and how the vibrations increased and the love was given back. The vegetables and herbs I grew vibrated with a holiness that was the life-force of God. Not only my family was reaping the benefit of that, but so was every living thing out my door. I watched the cycle of life. As the rabbits hid in their den, and ate my fresh lettuce, sometimes the hawks above would spot them and swooshed down for their lunch to feed their hatchlings. Sometimes the rabbits would escape, sometimes they were dinner, but it was always in balance, and life lived according to nature's rules.

Nature's schoolyard for me would be to watch the birds. I noticed the tenderness of the male cardinal feeding his mate, his beak intersecting with hers, and her coyness as to whether or not this was the right bird for her. He would come again and again if he was interested, and others would try, but not hard enough to win her. So she made her choice based on his behavior, and what her needs were, and they would set up a nest in a nearby tree. Building the nest together, other cardinal families would also nest nearby, and I never saw any wars between those birds.

Robins and bluebirds were also prevalent. Their melodious songs still sing in my heart. Their presence would to me, bring joy to the earth, and they always had enough, and so they sang. They sang no matter what. They always felt happy to me. Their singing resonated in a part of my soul that let me know it is always in divine right order, like a sunny blue day, or a cool breeze.

I would learn later of Icaros - divine songs of healing used in the Amazon to elucidate a feeling by having it dance out of the vibration of your soul. Sometimes it could dance in color, or with even a smell, shape or thought, but mostly through sound. I felt as though when the birds sang their song, they could dance that

vibration out of me to remind me of divine right order, as emmisaries of Spirit.

There was a strength abounding in these tiny creatures as well. Even if their nest was raided by one of the raccoons, or an owl, they still sang, but the song changed and they would fight. If another bird tried to get too close, mostly starlings or blue jays, as little as they were they could be quite ferocious, driving away much larger predators just with their energetic intent of protection, knowing that in turn, they too, were protected in the great web of life.

Some species would band together to drive away predators cooperatively. Hummingbirds would show me how ferocious a tiny little being could be if his or her loved one or home was threatened. They would dive-bomb and chase away what wasn't supposed to be there, like shamans driving out unwelcome spirits. These birds could do the impossible, with a combination of gentleness, beauty and inner strength that I have always admired.

It was during this wonderful time of intense spiritual

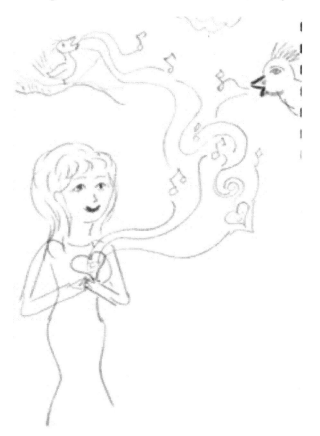

learning that I would sit and meditate and pray daily
for the Spirit to show me how to live. I believe I was
shown that through the birds and the trees. And one
spring day I was shown something more...

Mystic Awakening of an AmericanPhysician

It was a beautiful spring day, warm, sunny, and my twin boys, Derek and David, and I had a full morning of playing in the garden while their brothers were at school. When they would run too far, I would catch them by their little bib overalls, like little suitcase handles, at the back and they would squeal in excitement as they got 'caught' and got a 'ride' through the air. Sometimes I would carry them together one in each arm and they would laugh and laugh, as if it were the greatest thing in the world.

The peas were ready that day. Crisp and delicious, they went down like sugar.

"I like these Mommy!" said Derek.

"Me too!" chimed David.

We had lunch, cleaned up, and it was time for their nap. "But I don't wanna go to nap, I wanna play with my truck," said David.
"I wanna play with mine too!" said Derek.

Mystic Awakening of an American Physician
Linda Hostalek, D.O.

"No trucks, but you can bring your bunnies to bed," I said, "how would you like that?"

"Yeah!!!" they said together, in perfect harmony.

Those two taught me much about sharing, kindness, and trust. Being twins, they loved each other's company, and when shown a picture of the both of them they always pointed to the other and said "Me!" They truly could feel each other and had the most amazing bond. Because of this bond, they would climb out of their respective cribs, and continue to play together.

"Story Mommy, pleeeaaase??" Derek would ask.

"I love you Mommy," David would say, and then they would both start to sing in perfect harmony.

It was near their 2nd birthday and they were practicing singing the happy birthday song, only to themselves. "Happy birthday to me, happy birthday to me, happy birthday dear me-ee, happy birthday to me!"

Mystic Awakening of an AmericanPhysician

Since I needed to make sure they would sleep for the
structure of the household schedule, as well as my
own self-imposed schedule, I had taken to sitting at
the wall near the doorway. I rather enjoyed this.
Sometimes I would sing them to sleep, each one is
his own little bed, with blue and white comforters, and
a character alphabet theme on the wall. Today they
both began to sing to their stuffed little white furry
bunnies the birthday song. It got softer and softer
until the only sound was that of them quietly
breathing.

I had been praying and meditating while listening to
the birthday serenade. The soft beige carpet was
perfect for me to sit on in a lotus position against the
character and alphabet themed walls. Sometimes I
would read spiritual books during this time, and lately
I had been praying for Spirit to make Itself known to
me, to overcome any doubt I may have had.

I immersed myself in quiet reflection with my breath
when a great light came over me. I felt an opening in
my crown chakra, on the top of my head. It was

warm, and I had never experienced anything quite like this before. As I felt this presence open up my head, with a gentleness and strength, I felt the rest of my chakras become unzipped. First the crown, with a dazzling white light, danced through my body, opening my third eye, throat, heart, solar plexus, belly and pelvis all the way through me to the center of the earth. I was everywhere and nowhere at the same time. I was washed with liquid waves of love in every color imaginable - pinks, blue, purple white, yellow, gold, green, indigo, silver. They all danced throughout my body and throughout the universe. They danced into different geometric shapes that would change and change and change again, signifying to me the beauty and necessity of the change being the dance of life. It cannot stop, only change.

The undulating ribbons of colors bathed me with a knowingness that I was being purified, cleaned, and above all loved-- almost like I was being groomed for a spiritual task. It felt warm, like a warm river current, alive and electrifying, and it was pure love. This enveloping cocoon of liquid love showed me that all my needs will always be met, and that I am always taken care of in this great circle of life. Just like the trees and the birds and the plants, I too, am part of this wondrous spiritual world, more than just myself, or this planet, or humanity, but pure blissful spirit, one with all. I knew then deep into my essence, that the one I call God exists, and is pure love. I am so thankful for that experience.

To this day, I do not know if that took place over seconds, minutes or hours, for time truly did stand still and was seen for the illusion it truly is. Seeds were planted in me that day, and from that day on, I knew whatever I would face, I would be okay, although I could not have foreseen at that time just how much I would need that strength.

Late that night, from a window in the room just below Derek's and David's bedroom I watched the sky. I was still in awe of what had occurred earlier. As I looked up in thankfulness I saw those same types of lights in the sky - purple, green, blue, much fainter than what I had just experienced, but this was in this reality. I was mesmerized. I had just witnessed the northern lights, a rare occurrence for as far south as I was. It was another smile from God. "Thank you," I said.

Another jolt of color crossed the sky. I took it to mean "You're welcome."

I had great changes in my life after that, I began school, got divorced, experienced the whole cancer thing, got over it, graduated college, graduate school, medical school, and now I was ready for the next adventure...

Mystic Awakening of an AmericanPhysician

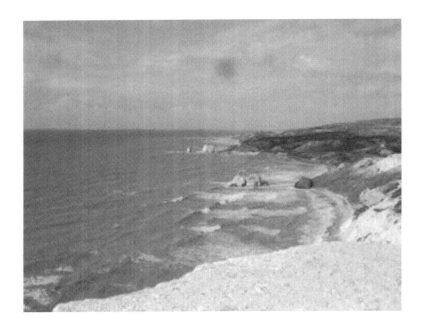

Chapter Three

Dreams from the Ether

The lecture by Richard, the shaman doctor, would be
on Friday night, that was only four nights away. I
began to get very excited about what this would mean
to me. It wasn't everyday that a picture would send
me off to the 'other' world, the world where time and
space stand still and great spiritual truths are
delivered in the most unusual way. I felt a calling in
my soul, a pulling that rational reality could not
explain. I knew this man was a key in my spiritual
growth. As I looked as his picture, his eyes
penetrated deep into my soul, and I began to dream.

Mystic Awakening of an AmericanPhysician

The first night I dreamt of him on a horse, he came to get me, also on a horse, to show me 'the way.' We crossed cavernous treacherous trails, steeped in mist, overlooking deep valleys below, and lush green mountains at eye level. He didn't say a word, but motioned me to come with him across the mountain top, across to the next 'world.' I went, and felt the strength and power of the mountain, as we blended into it, with an orgasmic warmth throughout my body as we merged, the mountain holding us, as we turned into stars. We then were in space. I woke up.

"Wow," I thought, this is going to be some ride. I felt strangely close to this man, as if we had just had a deep spiritual experience together. "That's crazy," I thought to myself, but as I thought that, I remembered an experience that happened to me about a year prior.

I had been accepted to go on a medical mission trip to Guatemala. I was very excited. I had always longed to learn more about the Mayan people, as their culture, what little I knew of it fascinated me. I could feel the power when I looked at their temples, or their

Mystic Awakening of an AmericanPhysician
Linda Hostalek, D.O.

hieroglyphs. We were to go to the highlands to help the indigenous Mayan poor who had very little access to medical care. It would be a trip of a lifetime. I got school credit to go, and a sponsor to fund my trip. My kids would stay with their dad. All was well to go. We would leave in late February and return back in two weeks in mid-March.

Around the first of the year I began to have dreams. Some dreams are just dreams, and some dreams come to us to teach us stuff. This was one of those dreams. I was high in the sky, laying down on a hard surface. The surface was made of stone, like a platform, in the middle of the sky. Fire burned in cauldrons around me, to illuminate me on this platform, like I was an offering or a gift. On this stone platform in the sky, behind me was an opening to a small room, a temple opening, things were kept there, although I did not know exactly what.

I had the sense of others around me, although I could not see anyone just yet. As I lay on this stone platform, I noticed I was lying naked, on my back, with hands grasping my ankles gently, but firmly, spreading

Mystic Awakening of an AmericanPhysician

my legs completely open while I laid on a soft spotted skin. My shoulders and arms were similarly held in place by invisible hards. As I looked down across my body. I watched the firelight flicker off my breasts, my belly, and my thighs. My naked body was decorated with beaded ropes of beautiful shells and stones and there were all kinds of flowers surrounding me. My vagina glistened and was engorged with anxious anticipation. I watched as light brown male hands caressed my full breasts and pink, erect nipples, fondling them with energetic intensity. His hands then moved to my belly and hips, touching them masterfully with deep concentration, making me melt in anticipation of what would happen next. He then stroked my thighs and held open my knees, I looked up to see whose hands they were. I saw a man in a full faced mask made up of smooth stones; blue, black and green, with gold around the eyes. His headdress was full of long dark green feathers, forming a full circle around his mask-face. He wore a cloak of jaguar skin, held together over his broad muscular chest with large clunky jewelry made of gold in large circles, triangles and squares with abalone inserts. His chest was partially covered with

Mystic Awakening of an AmericanPhysician
Linda Hostalek, D.O.

alternating layers of bones and weavings of some

sort.   As I looked in his eyes, we became one in an

orgasmic transmission of knowingness.   I was being

penetrated with knowledge, an initiation of some sort,

in the most pleasant of ways.

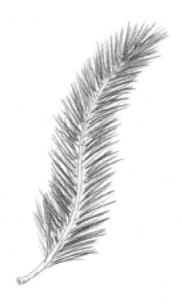

This wonderful dream was dreamt every night for

almost 3 months, each time exquisitely pleasant, but

also healing, and preparing me for something

grander. Every night the same masked man would

come and impart knowledge through me sexually,

while showing me secrets of the stars. He showed me how they swirl through the sky like an eddy in the ocean or the spiral of a nautilus shell, and how we humans were part of that same whole. I was shown how the sun throws spirals off, and how some can harm a planet such as earth, or keep it in place and protect it. The microcosm and the macrocosm had the same essential geometric design of life. A deep stirring in me knew I was being prepared to receive, and receive I did every night.

I knew at that time a man named Jeff. He was a protestant priest who had a wonderful, angelic smile and a head of sandy blonde hair and caring blue eyes. A handsome man, he was recently divorced and we became good friends. His wife had left him for a woman, and he was devastated and trying to get on with his life, and to live in his new reality. We had many conversations about God, timing, and synchronicity.   When I told him of my trip he said "I was called to give you $400 dollars. You must take it for your trip."

I was stunned. "Are you sure? What is this for?"

Mystic Awakening of an AmericanPhysician
Linda Hostalek, D.O.

"You"ll know what it was for when the time comes, but you need to take it."

"Thank you," I said, still a bit stunned that that much money was given to me out of the blue.

The vivid dreams were still occurring every night, and now, almost 3 months later, it was time to leave for Guatemala. There were about 20 of us and we met about 40 more docs and students that came from all over the United States. We flew into Guatemala City, and made our way via bus to Antigua, the former capital of Guatemala, before an earthquake devastated that area and the capital was moved to Guatemala City.

Antigua is a beautiful old city with cobblestone streets and colorful houses. Dogs roamed freely about the city square, with its street vendors and beautiful fountains. We stayed in a small hotel, just a block off the city center. We would stay there until everyone arrived the next day. As I was shown my room, which I would share with 2 other students, I noticed the sunset. Purples, pinks and blues shone over an ancient church with a cross and bell-tower in shadow. Vines had overgrown the brick structure, but it was still standing. Nature always wins.

The beauty of that moment struck me, the colors were amazing, and in the shadowy vista of the nighttime sky, a volcano was mildly erupting in the distance with an orange glow. Occasionally, it would sputter yellow fire out the reddish orange top, as the lava flowed down the side. Once in a while you could even hear the crackling of the lava with the explosions. It sounded like crisped rice cereal popping.

It was a long day, so I went to sleep, and arose the next day. No dreams of the impregnation of knowledge. Okay, I thought, and went about my day. We packed up on a bus and headed for a small convent in the Guatemalan highlands where we prepared a makeshift clinic. We stayed in a room with several beds and one very cold shower! We worked hard that week, seeing hundred of people, many of whom had not seen a doctor for many years.

Mystic Awakening of an AmericanPhysician
Linda Hostalek, D.O.

Some walked for over a week, many with bare feet, just to see us. This was a reality check for sure. I saw children with AIDS, many gynecological issues and neuro-fibro-matosis, a non-cancerous growth that can become horribly disfiguring. All things that were rarely, if ever, seen in a typical medical practice in the states.

I became very humbled at my surroundings. Although these people seemed very poor by our western standards, they were extremely rich in culture and spirit. Each person wore beautiful hand-crafted clothing, with elaborate embroidery and weavings. Different villages were distinguished by their colors in their weavings, and each one I encountered had a faith in the divine that made their lot in life not just tolerable, but joyful. I pondered the differences in our cultures, and just soaked it in.

Cars were rare. Most people got by on foot or donkey. The men all had machetes on their sides, and women carried their babies, sometimes 2 at a time, in their weavings on their backs, or in a nursing position if very young. The gratitude these people showed for even the smallest thing, like a pencil, was overwhelming. I fell in love with every one of them.

Down the street from the convent was a shrine to St. Simeon, and a traditional Mayan healer who did healing down the street in a small building. I snuck off with two others to go see what this was, as the nuns had forbade us from going there, thinking that that was the devil's magic. One of them, David, was no stranger to Guatemala. He had been coming here yearly for over ten years now. As we walked down the dirt road leading to the small, adobe brick structure, I bought some flowers and came to see the process. I was confused, as I saw alters with flowers, tobacco and alcohol as supplications for healings. The energy was divine and warm, and I felt no malice or malevolent intent. There was a line, one would go into this small room, lay your offerings next to the candles (there were many), get a blessing from the shaman, and exit out the other door.

I walked in following David, laid the flowers down and walked past the smoky alter to the man at the front of the room. He was a small, thin, brown man, dressed

Mystic Awakening of an AmericanPhysician
Linda Hostalek, D.O.

in traditional clothing, with a rattle, a rolled cigarette, and a bottle of aromatic liquid. As I walked by, I stopped, not knowing what to do, and he held out his hand, indicating to me to hold still, and he took that bottle, put it to his lips, and spat it out on me! Then he motioned me to turn around and he spat on me again! He took a long drag off his cigarette, and blew the smoke over me, front and back, rubbing it around my belly, heart and head. I was then motioned to move on and exit the building. I felt really good, lighter somehow, but I was really confused. In my world, we don't blow smoke on people or spit-- it would be considered very rude, but here, it seemed perfectly normal to everyone.

"What was that?" I asked David.

"Oh, the spitting?" he laughed. "That's the traditional way of cleansing. Smoke clears the energy off the centers, and the fire water or flower water cleans the aura. It's a little different than you're used to, huh?"

"It sure is."

Mystic Awakening of an AmericanPhysician

We ran back to the casa, the convent, for dinner.
We'd be in big trouble from the madre, the head
mother, if she knew we went there.

We were informed after the first couple of days that
we would have three days off-duty at the end of the
week. There were a couple of options if people
wanted to see some sites. That was a pleasant
surprise for me. I thought we were just mostly going
to work the whole time. There were trips to Lake
Atitlan, to Honduras to scuba dive, or to the black
sand beach, but the one that caught my eye was the
one to Tikal, one of the largest excavated Mayan
ruins. It was in the jungle, and I had always wanted to
go to the jungle, and, it cost $400. I knew I was
supposed to go there, that's what Jeff's spirit was
telling him when he gave me that $400. "Thank you
Jeff," I said silently .

After a small puddle jumper plane, we arrived in the
jungle of northern Guatemala. We were driven to a
small hotel on the grounds of the ruins. We were told
if we wanted to we could get up early, and had heard
that some people climb the pyramid number four just

before dusk to watch the sunrise. It was the tallest pyramid, and outfitted with railings and an observation deck that was perfect to watch the sun rise as you could see the entire complex, including the great jaguar pyramid from its summit. That sounded neat enough to get up early for! Six of us went on that side trip; my roommate, Carly, and I met the other four before light. We had flashlights with us, and raincoats, because it was raining. Through the dark and the rain, we heard growls, scary, loud utterances, and as we flashed our lights in the brush, all we saw were eyes. It was very unnerving. I would later find out that those were howler monkey, known for their fierce growls and equally fierce teeth. We walked and walked and probably got turned around about ten times. The map didn't make sense. We were beginning to wonder if we should turn back and wait for it to be light. After a few more growls from the forest, everyone else, except Carly and I, turned back. We then walked a little while longer, and saw a clearing.

"I think we've found it!" said Carly.

Mystic Awakening of an AmericanPhysician

"I think so too!" I said excitedly, "Let's climb it!"

"OK!"

So we climbed this tall, steep Mayan pyramid, in the jungle, in the rain, in the dark. I thought we must be crazy, but really didn't care. I was already wet, and the rain began to let up substantially. We climbed and climbed and climbed. This was one tall pyramid. We had to go slow because the tall, steep steps were very slippery. We held on to the edges as we climbed. We both sighed a sigh of relief when we hit the top. The rain turned into a drizzle, and the sun began to peek over the horizon.

I noticed a whole pavilion in front of us, and another, equally tall pyramid facing us. I breathed a prayer of thanksgiving to the creator for this wonderful moment. With each breath I felt more and more gratitude, for all my multitude of blessings-- for just being here! Only by the generosity of others was I here. I felt I was called here and cleansing was stirring in my soul. I was home. I opened my eyes, and now I could see where I was. I was at the stone platform in the sky

Mystic Awakening of an AmericanPhysician
Linda Hostalek, D.O.

with the temple on top, the place I'd dreamed about for months! I was god-smacked. We were on the jaguar pyramid in the jungle in Tikal!

I learned a lot that day. As we walked through the jungle after climbing down, I saw more birds than I had ever seen before. It was still early in the morning and I saw blue turkeys and pink spoonbills. I realized that growl that sounded like a jaguar was the sound of howler monkeys, now perched in the trees.

We toured the complex afterwards, seeing many temples, houses, and ball-courts. Mayan columns, also known as stelae, were everywhere, as well as frescos and reliefs. Each one fascinated me, as if I had been there in a previous life, and after the earlier experience, I was convinced by now that it was true.

I saw one particular temple that intrigued me. It was the temple of the sun, and one of the most special temples on the complex. The guide was explaining how the Mayan people lived their lives by both the lunar and solar calendars. There was a relief, or picture, of a sun face on the left side of the doorway.

Mystic Awakening of an AmericanPhysician

It was a fresco painted on an outer wall of a large face in a three dimensional relief, with rounded cheeks, and a strange open smile. I was mesmerized by the magnetic pull that sun face had on me. It appeared to me that the sun's eyes were looking right at me! Then, without warning, a pebble-sized piece of the temple relief shot off the temple itself, hitting me on my ankle! I reached down and picked it up. Made of clay, it had the yellowish fresco on one side. I slipped it into my pocket, and kept it.

After the tour, we went to the place where the small replica of the complex was. There was a mural depicting the shamans in that area. The chief wore a headdress of green feathers of the quetzal bird, a bird native to the area, and a cape of a jaguar! I would find out later that Tikal was famous for its jaguar shamans. This was a day that would live in my memory forever, teaching me energetically that all things are interconnected, and that gratitude is a manifesting force for good.

Mystic Awakening of an AmericanPhysician
Linda Hostalek, D.O.

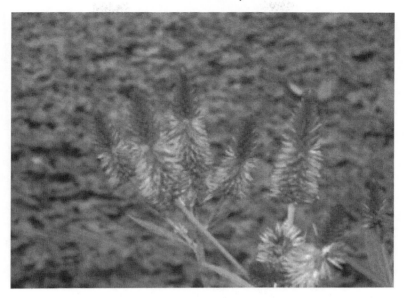

Mystic Awakening of an AmericanPhysician

Chapter Four

Synchronicity

Life felt more synchronistic after that experience. My
aura felt lighter and I felt spiritually 'cleaner' and
lighter. I would often visit Guatemala in my dreams
and began to learn a little about shamanism through
reading books on the subject. I felt very much in tune
with the jaguar, the primal feline. This was how I was
being tapped by the vibration of life that would lead
me in different directions to learn things for my higher
knowledge. I was learning to listen to the voice of
spirit. Because of this increase in my awareness, I
was excited to wonder what could happen with this
shaman on the back of the magazine when I would
meet him at the Blue Feather. Would he be a new
teacher, or was I being led there for a different
reason? Whatever it was, it was strong and profound.

Mystic Awakening of an AmericanPhysician

I was ready to listen, and I began to have more dreams.

The dreams of this new shaman doctor were not sexual, but sensual and intriguing. I felt a type of pulling into unity with him-- and I had not yet even met this man! I began to feel shifting in my energy fields during dreamtime with this man. Dark ribbons of oily substances came out of my energy body, especially in the lower centers-- I was being cleaned! How odd I thought, but life being what it was, I was thankful I was being shown methods of healing. This blended well with what I had seen in the hospitals, and I felt clearer and cleaner each day I awoke.

Friday finally arrived, and I drove to the Blue Feather bookstore to the 'Intro to Peruvian Shamanism' class. I paid my fee, and sat down on the floor and listened. Rhonda, the host, introduced Richard, a physician, shaman, healer, author, and teacher. He was a handsome man, in his late thirties, about 6 foot tall, of sturdy build, with deep hazel eyes. His sandy brown hair was pulled back in a ponytail, and he wore a wide striped hooded shirt with a single front pocket, dark cargo pants with lots of pockets, and brown hiking boots.

He noticed me right away, and when his eyes met mine, an electrical sensation linked us immediately. We had already known each other on a very deep spiritual level.

I listened as he spoke of the ancient culture of the Inca people, the Q'ero, who still live in the sacred valley in Peru. He had studied for years under his mentor, the wonderful Jose Luis, and was so moved by the spiritual healings and lifestyle that he had given up traditional medicine. Now, with permission of the elders, he taught traditional Incan shamanism.

He introduced us to the concept of the three energetic centers of the body, the belly, the heart and the head, which correspond to the three worlds: the ukhupacha, or underworld, corresponded to the belly; the kaypacha corresponded to this world and the heart; and the hannapacha, or heavenly realm, was associated with the head. He spoke of serpents, jaguars, and condors, and of the holy places in Peru that resonated with those animistic energies.

I had waited for this my whole life! I wanted to learn more. My body vibrated with the knowingness that this was right for my path. He came up to me after the talk and said he had dreamt of me, and asked if I had some time to go have a drink. We went to a restaurant down the block, and began to talk. He was intrigued with me and I with him.

We walked to a restaurant a couple of doors away. Mediterranean in theme, it was a bit dark, but a wonderful place to go and have a chat. "So," I asked, "What led you into shamanism?"

"I had everything a person would want: money, a beautiful wife, a nice big home, a high paying and respectable profession, but I just wasn't happy." He looked away, as though to relive that aspect of life momentarily, and then said "I was relaxing in my pool, and I thought there has to be more than this. I had reached the top of the mountain, but I was not fulfilled. So I thought I would climb real mountains."

Mystic Awakening of an AmericanPhysician
Linda Hostalek, D.O.

"Is that when you went to Peru?" I asked.

"Not at first." Richard went on, "I had heard of a man named Jose Luis, a shaman, who grew up at the base of Machu Picchu. I knew a friend, who knew a friend, etc. It came to pass that we met, and we instantly connected, kinda like you and me."

"Really?"

"Well, maybe a little a different." he chuckled. "But I do feel this amazing connection between us." His eyes became serious as he said, "I have dreamt of you, and now you are here. The question is now, why?"

"I saw the magazine with your picture of you on the horse in the mountains. I knew I had to meet you, that there was something there, that you had something to teach me." I felt a bit split, as I was intrigued with this man's knowledge, yet there was a very magnetic attraction between us, and I wanted to keep this professional, although my heart pounded. "Do you go to Peru very often?" I blurted out. "I have always wanted to go to Peru, especially Machu Picchu."

"I go there every few months now. I have made some good friends there, and have been privileged enough to spend time in the villages. Jose Luis has arranged for some of us to go to the mountains. We bring western medicine and they teach us their ways. We help support the school and the children, and it is absolutely beautiful, the whole experience."

"Is that where you had your picture taken?" I asked.

Richard laughed and said, "It took three days by horse or mule just to get there! That was my horse for the duration of the trip. It can be pretty rough. We're going again in a few weeks."

My eyes got wide as saucers, "Any chance that I could come with?"

"Can you ride a horse?"

"Yes I can."

Mystic Awakening of an AmericanPhysician
Linda Hostalek, D.O.

"Well I'd have to clear it, not just anyone can do that, It's pretty intense. If this were to actually occur, I'd have to clear it with the others, and teach you some things quick to bring you up to speed about the Q'ero and some of their customs."

"I would have to clear it with my school, and my rotation." I said as my mind raced furiously. "If it is meant to be, it will all come together. I can't tell you how much I would like to do this trip." I went on "I have been to Ecuador and Guatemala on medical mission trips, and I'm sure I could help and that I would learn a lot too. And since you're a doctor, you could be my mentor, if you would be okay with that."

"Usually I wouldn't even consider it, but I did dream of you, and not just once or twice, so I'll run it by the others, and we'll see."

I couldn't help but smile. We talked a bit about his previous trips, and some of my energetic experiences. There was a reason I felt so magnetically attracted to this man through his picture. The possibility of actually going to Peru was almost completely absurd, yet felt so right.

We parted the restaurant, and as he gave me a hug, our electrical energies rushed together. We made plans to get together in a couple of days to begin my 'training' because we would be with indigenous people and I needed to at least have a basic understanding of their culture if this would come to pass. He would contact his colleagues, and I my school, and I would see about the logistics of my life, kids, school stuff, how to pay for it, etc. It seemed improbable, but the energy searing through me said otherwise.

Everything worked out extremely easily, almost magically. I was allowed the time off to go, although no credit would be given to me. But I didn't care-- I was going to go on a medical mission trip to Peru!! I was so excited. I had read books on shamanism, and even though I was going there to work, I just knew that just being in the presence of those holy mountains would change me forever.

Mystic Awakening of an AmericanPhysician
Linda Hostalek, D.O.

We met several times over the next couple of weeks. We walked in the forest and felt the energies there. His dog, Dexter, would often accompany us and our energies became more and more familiar together, as if we were destined to be there right then in the presence of the forest. He spoke of mountain spirits, mountain 'angels' or 'Apu's' and how holy they were in the Incan tradition. We would see some of them on our trip. "Each Apu has its own personality, its own job description," he said. "We make offerings, called despachos for thanksgiving to the mountain, and also for permission to be there, for its blessing."

"What is a despacho?" I asked, beaming with excitement.

"It is basically an offering. You take a piece of paper, and put your prayers in it with coca leaves, red and white carnations to represent earth and sky, corn, beans, seeds, incense, candy, all kinds of stuff goes into one of those. Each one represents something different. There are despachos for thanksgiving, for blessings, for new beginnings, to help someone cross over, and even some to turn away sorcery. They sell kits in Peru that have all the items in them, it makes it very convenient."

"That sounds like a very nice ceremony."

Richard said "It is very nice. The rituals of this body of medicine are very nice, but you have to earn the rites. You cannot just receive them; you have to do the ceremony and the work. You have to compile a mesa, get rites handed down to you, and learn how to utilize your medicine body for the good of all."

"What is a mesa?" I asked. I felt like a three year old with all my questions, but I just wanted to learn all that I could.

"A mesa is a bundle that contains your cuellas, your special stones that you work with until you have a relationship with them. It becomes a living altar, a portable altar that will become very special to one who resonates with this medicine. We won't have much time to compile a mesa while we are there, but when we come back to the states, you will learn to compile your own mesa."

Mystic Awakening of an AmericanPhysician
Linda Hostalek, D.O.

That sounded good. For the past few years, the concentration of my energy focus was around Pinky, my vogel crystal. I took several crystal classes through the people at the Cranial Academy, and had learned quite a lot about their energies, and how to use them to do healings. I didn't use her (Pinky) much to do healings, but mostly for personal meditations, and to concentrate on my studies. I had learned from my time at Argonne national lab and the Cranial Academy about the various properties of crystals and I was attuning myself to their vibrations.

We would do ceremony in the woods. I would take out Pinky, and Richard would take out his mesa, and we would bathe them in the sun. He took a piece of palo santo, a type of peruvian wood that was used as incense, and put the smoke around the crystal, his mesa, and over our luminous body, or aura. He would have me stand and he took the smoking stick and cleansed me by blowing the incense over me with a feather. First my feet, then legs, belly, heart, head, then turned and did the same, then I held my arms out and he did the sides of my body, then the top of my head, and I would do the same to him. It smelt woody fresh, yet clean and the vibration changed from normal to spiritual. He would then rattle and invite me to go inward to those centers he talked about in the workshop, around the belly, heart and head via the serpent, jaguar and condor, as he sprayed the same type of aromatic liquid over me that the Mayan shaman did in Guatemala.

"Feel the vibration of Pacha-mama, mother earth, and also Wiracocha, father sky" said Richard as he rattled. "Go deeper." He taught me a crash course in basic shamanism 101, in those quick weeks. We became closer, and the connection grew. He was a patient teacher, and very kind. I looked forward to my one-on-one lessons.

****Amaru, the serpent****

I began to have dreams again. During this time, the forms of the dreams were Richard giving me lessons, showing me the urupacha. The serpent, Amaru, the animistic archetype of the lower realm, was spiraling in my belly, eating any leftover darkness and showing me the potential of my dreams. Because I had wanted to go to Peru and study shamanism, the teacher appeared, and I had manifested the circumstances to allow this to happen. The blockages to prevent this manifestation were also removed.

****Chocochinkay, the jaguar****

In another dream, I was a jaguar, waking up; Richard was also a jaguar, and we explored the mountains and jungles, and as we did, I noticed a warmth in my heart growing. This was the kaypacha, this realm, represented by the chocochinkay, the jaguar, in the heart realm of this reality. I learned that we are all pure love in our purest form. Sensual and dreamy, these were the pleasures of life.

*****Apuchin, the condor****

In another, I was a flying condor, overseeing my entire life, how it had been laid out to get to where I was now. I would switch into being a hummingbird occasionally, but the flying was very fast, and in my vision I could see all the way to outer space-- there were no limits. This was shown to me to be

Mystic Awakening of an AmericanPhysician

representative of the hannapacha, the heavenly
realm, and the animistic archetype of this realm is
Apuchin, the condor.

Richard was very cognizant of my dreams. He would
call me and ask about my dreams, and fill in details
that only the dreamer would know. They were my
lessons. This was a deep connection of a spiritual
encounter that touched me in the same way that Spirit
did when it came into me when the kids were little in
their bedroom, and also the dreams of the jaguar
shaman. I was always able to listen to animals, and
now that seemed especially important, along with
listening to plants and observing the signs in the
clouds.

There was one other dream of note, which occurred
after the three worlds were shown to me. In that
dream, I was in a very verdant, green mountain
setting. The mountains were so tall that all you saw
was space, mist and green mountains. I was on top
of a mountain looking over the side.

Mystic Awakening of an AmericanPhysician
Linda Hostalek, D.O.

I flew around a while, and turned into a condor again. Then I landed and ran further up the mountain as a jaguar, where I turned and looked back over my shoulder where I saw a cave. I shape-shifted into a serpent and slithered in to the cave to explore. There were energies there of ancient peoples and other worlds. I didn't know quite what to make of it, but I noticed three distinct spirals, which seemed to glow. The glowing indicated to me to pay attention to those spirals, and that they were important.

Then I was in my own bed in my own room, still in dreamtime, and I saw Richard hovering over my bed. He carried those three spirals on his luminous body, and he began to make love to me. With each thrust, the spirals was transferred from his luminous field to mine. After a period of intense thrusting, an orgasmic transfer took place of all three spirals at once. The spirals were now imprinted onto me. I was playing in a whole new territory now.

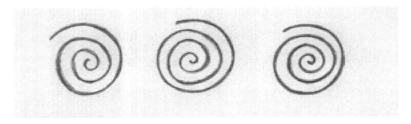

The day had finally arrived. I kissed my kids goodbye and off I went. I met up with Richard and we left for the thirty-six hour travel to Cuzco. We took a cab to the airport, and had a very long line to wait in for our international flight to Lima. "How was dreamtime last night?" He asked with knowingness in his eyes. We moved slowly closer in the international line waiting to enter the airport terminal. His cell phone rang. It was one of his colleagues, Jorge, from Peru.

"We have to leave for camp today," he said. "If we don't leave, the trails will be washed out, there is a huge storm forecast. So we won't be able to wait for you, sorry."

"Okay, will anyone be going later?" Richard asked.

Mystic Awakening of an AmericanPhysician
Linda Hostalek, D.O.

"No, we're all leaving today, we'll be back at the regular time, but there's no way any of us can wait around or we won't be able to get up there."

He looked at me and said "The others are leaving for camp today, there's a big storm coming, and in Peru in the mountains, when it rains there can be mudslides, and then you have to wait a long time to be able to pass. The question is, do we still go?"

I was heartbroken; all this had come together in such a magical way, only to possibly not even happen now. I moved my suitcase further down the queue.

"We can still go, you know," he said, "I know my way around there pretty good."

"Where will we go, where will we stay?" I asked.

"Trust me?" he asked with a sparkle in his eye.

"Yes," I said, Spirit had led me this far, and by now, I truly did trust him.

Mystic Awakening of an AmericanPhysician

"Good," he smiled, playfully, "do you want to go?"

"Yes, I do!" I said.

And so we went.

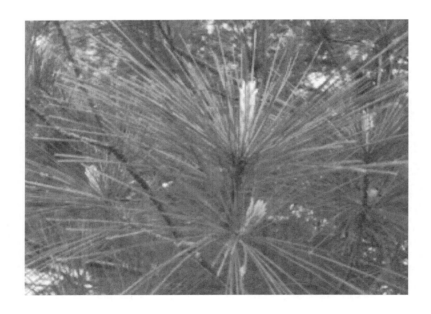

Chapter Five

Cuzco surprise

It was a very long day and night. We boarded our
plane in Chicago for Miami, and then had a layover
until about midnight, when we boarded for Lima. I
was tired, and fell asleep on his shoulder in the
crowded economy section. It felt safe and
comfortable. I could sense his energy, and he and I
both fell into a comfortable, cuddly rest. We arrived in
Lima, went through customs, and waited around
again to catch our flight to Cuzco. Thirty-six hours
later, we arrived.

Although I was very tired, the sight of Cuzco for the
first time was magical. There were vendors in the

airport parking lot selling colorful blue, green and
white bags of coca leaves. Festival music played in
the background, and the beeps of cars and buses and
the bustle of the tourist hustle joined the symphony of
sounds. The air was moist and warm, and the sun lit
up the entire city while the smell of diesel fuel
permeated the air.

We grabbed our luggage, and took a taxi to the city
square. The fountain splashed in the middle, while
beautiful trees shaded benches that lined the
sidewalks. Old cathedrals flanked the square, as did
shops, restaurants, and some places to stay. We
walked around the square, and found a small wooden
doorway that led to a long hall. It was a hotel,
although you wouldn't know it from the front. The
man asked us what kind of room we wanted, regular
or matrimony. We were so tired, I really didn't care at
that point, and I just wanted to sleep. The lack of
sleep, and now the high mountain air was starting to
get to me, and all I could think about was a shower,
and some sleep.

Mystic Awakening of an AmericanPhysician
Linda Hostalek, D.O.

We were given a key and led to a courtyard. There were three floors, and the staircase to reach the floors was through this courtyard. There were flowers growing, and the sunlight filtered in from above like a picture. We trudged up the three flights of stairs, weary from lack of sleep and the high altitude. We finally arrived at our room. We opened the dark, old, wooden door, and there we were. The room was small, with one bed, a chair, and a small bath, barely fitting in the small space. We looked at each other, and the repressed sexual tension between us erupted.

Suddenly I wasn't tired anymore! We both dropped our bags on the floor as we embraced and enjoyed our first delicious kiss, closing the door behind us with our bodies. Passionately, we undressed each other revealing ourselves as we headed for the shower. He had tattoos of his power animals under his clothing, and now I got to enjoy them; a bear, a wolf, a hummingbird and a jaguar, I enjoyed each one thoroughly as I explored his naked body with the voracious appetite of a feline in heat. We lingered under the warm, wet, water dripping down our soapy bodies, and we caressed each other and made sure every part of us was clean. We made love over and over and finally we fell asleep in each other's arms.

When we awoke later that day, we went to have something to eat. I felt rather light-headed when I was upright. I wasn't used to the altitude. "Here, drink this," Richard instructed, "It will make you feel better." He handed me coca tea, a staple in the Andean culture. "You need to eat." He ordered us breakfast in Spanish. Although it was late in the day, he convinced them to make us eggs, huevos rancheros. They were delicious. He made some phone calls, and then we walked around the square a bit, the Plaza de Armes, stopping frequently in the thin air.

"I see some of my friends, let me introduce you," he said to me. We arrived to a table on the open air in the square. The table was very dark wood, loaded with tortilla chips and salsa, and a variety of drinks.

"Come join us Ricardo!" said one.

Mystic Awakening of an AmericanPhysician
Linda Hostalek, D.O.

"Who's your friend?" asked another.

We sat for a while and exchanged some casual
conversation, although it was mostly in Spanish, and I
didn't understand a lot of the conversation. We were
with three men, Eduardo, Alberto, and Francisco,
remaining members of the shaman network that Jose
Luis used to work with. He had recently parted ways
due to a difference in value systems that revolved
around teaching the Incan ways. They were talking
about Jose Luis, why they parted and where he was
now. He was on an expedition in the mountains, and
would not be back for a week or more. He was not
with the others on the mountain mission trip. These
three men were also shamans, and led many people
in training of the medicine path in Peru. They all knew
each other very well. Eduardo and Alberto had
recently come back from a pilgrimage to one of the
holy mountains, Ausangante, and were now enjoying
piso sours, a common drink in Peru. Richard had one
too, but the thought of alcohol made my stomach stir,
so I ordered another coca tea instead.

Mystic Awakening of an AmericanPhysician

We returned to our hotel and made love some more, and when we woke up the next day Richard said, "Your training begins today."

"OK," I said jubilantly.
We walked all over Cuzco that day. We went to the traditional side of town. Past the old Inca walls, past the restaurants and shops, the terrain changed from commercial and touristy to a more like a neighborhood. There was a large, tall archway that separated the two sections. Through this archway, the vibration changed. There were open shops everywhere, full of exotic colors, smells and sounds.

We were looking for traditional weavings in the Q'ero style, often used for mesa cloths. We passed hundreds in every color and style imaginable. He taught me to look for those made of alpaca, as now many vendors were making them out of polyester, some even machine made, and that would not contain the same energy as that made from alpaca, especially if it was old, and contained the energy of the previous owner. He showed me how to bite the cloth, and to check for the springiness that only a natural material can provide. He also told me to smell it; there should be a characteristic naturally pleasant odor. You could tell the signs of true alpaca weavings that way. In addition to the material, the design was also important. He taught me to look for certain patterns in the weavings that represented mountains, although to me they looked like stylized 'x's. He explained, "The Q'ero live in a vertical reality. Their concept of life is very different from ours in the west. Those represent mountains, as seen from above."

This culture did indeed live in a different way than I was used to; it was much closer to what I had seen in the Guatemalan highlands than in the USA. I eventually bought a traditional mesa cloth, with red and black woven bands, stitched together with a red yarn. Some of the bands had black 'mountains' on red, and other bands had red 'mountains' on a black background. There were some other colors woven in there, brown, yellow and orange, as well, although they were less predominant.

Next we went to the 'witch' market, the market that the locals came to buy 'cures,' and florida water, also known as 'agua de florida'. "Florida water is a staple in peruvian shamanism. It's made from the essence of flowers steeped in water that has never seen light. The water comes from an underground spring, a holy spring, called a pacarina," Richard stated. "This helps to clear the aura, and is good for cleansing space."

There were lots of interesting things in that store. There were beads and shells, dolls, little miniatures of all kinds of stuff; houses, animals, furniture, people. The shelves had many wrapped packages wrapped in newspaper. There were rattles, bells, and long strips of individually wrapped candy, also in miniature people, men and women, houses, etc. "What are those for?" I asked as I pointed to the miniature candies wrapped in strips.

"Those are for despachos, those offerings I told you about earlier. We are going to do a despacho today, so you'll get to see then." He then proceeded to order in Spanish some of those newspaper wrapped bundles. Turns out those are despacho kits.

Mystic Awakening of an AmericanPhysician
Linda Hostalek, D.O.

Complete except for flowers and coca leaves. We would get those from different vendors.

I found a box of rattles and picked them up one by one, and began to rattle them. I found one that I liked, and it felt good in my hand. "I like this one," I said.

"It works for you, are you going to get it?" Richard asked.

"Yeah, I think so. It feels good."

I purchased the rattle, some palo santo, and some florida water, and Richard purchased a large bag of items, including several despacho kits, several bottles of florida water and many bundles of palo santo. "You can't get this in the states, so I always stock up whenever I'm here," he said.

We passed many markets, full of flowers, clothing, tropical fruits, and goods of every kind. Freshly dressed birds hung from their feet with the blood still flowing out their neck, next to a stand selling boots or bags. Everyone had something to sell and it made the market a vibrant thriving place. We passed a stand manned by a very large Peruvian woman with double braids under her traditional black hat. She wore the typical clothing of a skirt, sweater, and criss-cross sandals. She was selling coca leaves in a huge bag, about three foot high, stuffed with coca leaves. They were fresh and green, pliable, and beautiful. You could buy them by the bunch, or by the bag. There were also little rocks being sold next to the big bag of leaves.

"Those are calcium carbonate, it helps to release the coca out of the leaves. That's why some people have poor teeth, they chew on the rocks too much." Richard enlightened me. "These are really fresh. In the Incan tradition, coca leaves are holy. In addition to being a great antidote for altitude sickness, they are used to make kintos, prayer offerings, which you will see later when we make our despacho. They are also used as gifts, and carpi, gifts of coca leaves, kintus of a type, to a friend. It's an honor if someone offers you a carpi. It is actually fed to you by another."

Mystic Awakening of an AmericanPhysician
Linda Hostalek, D.O.

He reached into the newly purchased bag of leaves, took three out, made a blessing over them with his breath, and put them in my mouth. "Chew," he said. I did. It was rather nice, although I had visions of chewing tobacco and wasn't sure what to do after they were finished (you spit them out).

The flower market was next. So many beautiful flowers in all colors, shapes and sizes, some I had never seen before. There were calla lilies in white, yellow and pink, bordered by roses, and multiple colored carnations. The scent was intoxicating! I was enjoying the moment as a hedonistic flower lover, when Richard began his teaching again. "Red and white carnations are what we need. Carnations hold the highest vibration of all the flowers, which is why you see it used in many spiritual traditions all over the world. The red represents the earth mother, Pachamama, and the white represents Wirachocha, the heavenly father, if you will. There are other flowers used for other reasons, but the most important and traditional are the red and white carnations, the blood of the mother, earth, and the clouds of the sky, heaven."

Mystic Awakening of an AmericanPhysician

We finished our shopping, and we began to head back to the other side of town. Just before we reached the archway that was the boundary, we stopped and bought a late lunch or early dinner. Simple, it was a small, round, baked potato on a stick, with a piece of grilled, steak-type red meat skewered on top. Meat on a stick, how wonderful! It was delicious. I wondered why we didn't have this in the states.

We unleashed our libidos as we unleashed our treasures, and then took a small nap before our next adventure. We were to take our purchases, the flowers, coca leaves, florida water, and the despacho kit to a special place to ask permission of the Apus to be here and to do our work, the work of my initiation into this sacred place. I brought my newly acquired mesa cloth, and brought Pinky, my vogel crystal, and wrapped her up in it.

Our driver drove us to a place about an hour away from Cuzco, I don't know where I was. It was late afternoon, and this mountain pass was not on the

usual tourist list. We were the only humans around.
There were ruins there, and we climbed inside the
perimeter of the remaining rock walls with three
windows still intact, and an open ceiling overhead. It
was God's cathedral. Richard opened up his mesa
and motioned for me to do the same with my cloth
wrapped around Pinky. He lit the palo santo and
cleansed our luminous fields. He spat florida water in
the different directions, expanding the luminous field
around us. He made bundles of three perfect coca
leaves, kintus, and placed them carefully in the
'windows.' He rattled his rattle and spat florida water
in each of the six directions and called out to spirit,
opening the sacred space around us.

I watched as his features transformed in front of me.
His handsome smiling face became serene and other-
world-like. He looked much older, like an ancient
medicine man with prominent features radiating
vibrational serenity and wisdom. "That process of
spitting is called camay," Richard said, "it infuses the
area with spirit."

Mystic Awakening of an AmericanPhysician

He then called on Pachamama, mother earth, to hold and protect us, on the four cardinal directions, and on the Great Spirit, Wiracocha, above. He rattled and we journeyed into the essence of the Andes around us. He then opened the despacho kit, revealing its cornucopia of treasures. I was delighted by the beautiful display of leaves, flowers, seeds, fruit, nuts, sweets, horoscopes, miniatures, rainbows and cloud representations that he formed into a spirit offering.

Part of the offering were bundles of coca leaves called 'kintus.' He took my hand and placed three coca leaves inside my palm. Smiling, he showed me how to make kintus by picking three perfect coca leaves and placing them in the correct position. The stems needed to be down, with the vein of the leaf to the back. He held my hand as I made my first proper 'kintu,' and he motioned to me to place it to my lips and blow my prayers and intent into the kintu. The group of three leaves would hold our prayers, and those prayers would go in to the despacho. We breathed our breath, called 'samay,' into the kintus to infuse them with our prayers. The flowers, in turn would also hold our prayers in the despacho. We prayed and rattled and prayed some more. Our

vibrations became unified with the beat, echoing the

heartbeat of the mountains.

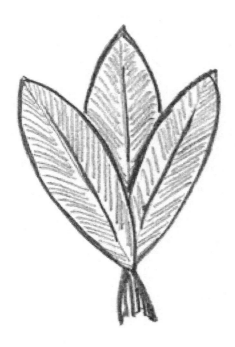

My prayer was for both seeking spiritual

enlightenment and learning from this wonderful place.

I wanted my heart to be pure, and my energy clean.

The transmission of energy, via our prayers with our

breath, provided our intent of respect, humility and

willingness to learn. I truly could feel the high spiritual energy of this place, called 'sami,' a harmonizing force. He made a fire and burnt the despacho while I looked away. "Its disrespectful to watch the spirits consume the offering while its being burned," Richard said as the spirits of that place enjoyed our offering. I turned my head, looking at the beautiful Andes mountains, taking in all the sami of this wonderful, spirit-filled place. The scent of the despacho filled the cool mountain air, enhancing the experience as I sat in silence, thanking the spirits.

When the burning was complete, we packed up our belongings. Still feeling in blissful harmony, I saw a sparkly small rock calling to me from the ground. It was a gift to me! I put that in my brand new 'mesa' - I had my first 'cuella,' or small stone that talked to me. We were accepted by the spirits, and more training would commence in the morning.

Mystic Awakening of an AmericanPhysician
Linda Hostalek, D.O.

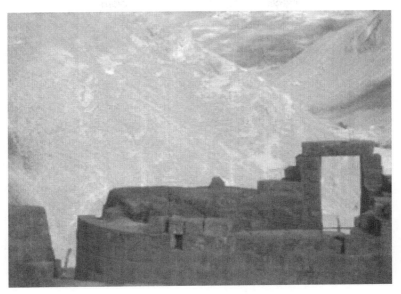

Mystic Awakening of an AmericanPhysician

Chapter Six

The Training Begins

In the center of Cuzco are the remains of an Inkan temple. In years past, the temple of the moon was covered in silver, and the temple of the sun was covered in pure gold. Conquistadors removed the precious metals during their occupation, sending it back to Spain. This ceremonial center was built over sacred ley lines, electro-magnetic energetic lines in the earth that hold special significance, like meridians of the earth. These ley lines form all over the earth, and indigenous peoples have built temples over these power places all over the world.

Mystic Awakening of an AmericanPhysician

A Catholic cathedral was built over the ruins. There is a dark Christ in the chapel of that church that is rumored to contain an Inkan mummy. It was common practice to mummify elders in ancient times, to keep their essence with those still living on earth. We toured the ruins and then sat in the chapel. I felt a presence opening my heart chakra as the eyes of the dark Christ met mine. I felt layers of previous pain and suffering melt off of me, as if it was never meant to be there in the first place. I finally understood the Catholic practice of keeping relics of saints for their essence. I was at peace. A knowingness encompassed my being as I was receiving the downloading of information from that Christ, but I was not yet ready to process all of it.

I learned that Cuzco was the ancient capital city of the Inca. The Spanish came in the mid-sixteenth century and took over the culture. Cuzco meant navel, as it was thought that Cusco is the navel of the earth, the center of the world. Sucsayhuaman was a large complex, with interlocking layers of giant blocks in a zig-zag pattern that some say represented the teeth of the head of the jaguar, while Cuzco represented the umbilicus. It was a ceremonial center and possibly a military fortress, but the blocks that it was built of were stunning. They were in three layers; again the number three is sacred in Incan cosmology, representing the three worlds, uru-pacha, kay-pacha, and hanna-pacha. Some were taller than two or more humans, but the joining space in between could not fit a blade of grass. They were irregular in shape, and tilted slightly in, most likely due to the frequent earthquake activity in this area. It was an architectural achievement that impressed me everywhere we went. Thrones built into the site where shamans welcomed the sun were carved into the rock, as was a ceremonial fountain.

There were remnants of ceremonial sites everywhere. One was a small, natural cave, a bit away from the main complex. "Let me show you this," Richard said. Inside this small cave was a small altar-like structure. There was a small window, from which you could see the complex. Being there was like being in the womb of the great mother herself. I found myself both giddy from the powerful vibrations, and humbled by them. This was where the lady of the mountain lived.

Mystic Awakening of an AmericanPhysician

Richard called it a moon cave. He smiled serenely as he drank in the essence of that place.

Kintus were everywhere inside that small cave, but no tourists. We took some time for prayers and did a small ceremony in there. I could feel the feminine energy welcoming us. I felt very happy, like this was a marker on my path. I was so grateful to be there and to exchange my energy with that of this place. It just felt so right, Pachamama holding me in her warm embrace.

As my spirit merged with the energy, I was transported in a mystical journey to deep in the earth, where I saw a snake smiling at me, as it swirled and ate its own tail as it happily danced. It turned into a crocodile/cayman type of creature and dove down into dark, murky waters. I felt a pulling presence in my belly similar to what I felt in the dreams previously with Richard. The energy went down my legs into my feet and into the earth through the soles of my feet.

Later, I would come to learn how important feet are in energy medicine. Like hands, the middle of feet channel the body's energetic centers, where the electromagnetic healing energy passes through. Healing hands can discharge enough electrical energy to be measured by modern means. When a healer heals, energy comes out of the hands to be the channel of the healing. When a person balances their energy with the earth, dense, heavy energy that needs to leave the body will often do so through the soles of the feet, similar to how lightning that strikes a person will find ground through the feet. As I came back into my body, I felt lighter and slightly disorientated, but I breathed and thanked the earth, Pachamama, for grounding me and cleansing me with her healing presence.

Later that day, I would come across a beautiful blue green stone, which called to me. I picked it up and I could see a brown man in a field next to a strong flowing river, picking up this stone as he plowed his field with a hand-tool. I saw blue, misty mountains in the back, behind the swift, flowing river, which I took to be the Urubamba. The very clear communication of the stone's vibrations led me to put it in my mesa, with its permission. My mesa was growing, as was my medicine body.

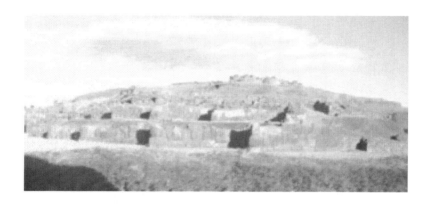

Chapter Seven

Opening My Heart

If Saysuhuaman was the head of the jaguar, then
Moray was the heart. Moray is a series of concentric
rings carved into a natural depression in the
landscape of the Andes mountains. Three sets of
rings (again three is a sacred number in Incan
cosmology) forming bowls of consciousness of the
plants that Pachamama nourished therein. Potatoes,
for example, are said to be over one thousand in
variety, many being developed by the ancients here.
Thought to be an agricultural center, as many different
altitudes are represented, the rings concentrated the
energetic field and magnified the ubiquitous field
energies present there.

Mystic Awakening of an AmericanPhysician

Richard and I traveled there to pay homage to the earth energies and spirits that reside there. It was a windy and overcast day, with the sun only occasionally peeking out to warm us. From the top of the mountain, you could see the rings as they reached deep down like a man-made collapsable cup, fully opened, each ring a little smaller than the one above, each filled with green vegetation that differed depending on which level you were on. We made sure we had plenty of water, and our ceremonial items (mesa, rattle, florida water, etc) and began the long, slow descent down. It took a long time to reach the circular bottom, but it was worth it. Looking up from the bottom, you could sense and see the care that had been put into this structure for many centuries. The energy concentrated with each concentric ring. That, coupled with the decrease in altitude, energized me. I loved this place!

The ground was rich with sparkly white and reddish brown, clay-like rocks that would crumble into a shimmery powder if squeezed. I put a large one in my backpack near the beginning of our descent because I thought it was so pretty, but it was a pile of powder by the time we got down to the bottom of the rings. As I opened up my backpack at the bottom of the rings, I saw the powder everywhere. I could hear Spirit's voice telling me that everything in this world crumbles eventually, that the only thing that matters is spirit, love. I felt that profoundly in my soul.

While I did not think in terms of greed when I picked up that beautiful rock and put it in my backpack, I felt a wave of shame fall over me when I realized that in my greed to keep the beauty of that rock with me, it vanished into a pile of sparkly powder. This showed me that the beauty in life may be fleeting, but the essence always remains. The sparkles that attracted me to the shiny rock were still there, although the form of beauty was different. I realized that sometimes it is better to drink in the life, the beauty of the moment, for it always changes and is never the same for long. Even something as seemingly stable as a rock or a planet can go away. Love is the only permanent thing, and that was evident everywhere, if I could only see!

Mystic Awakening of an AmericanPhysician

I took out my mesa, as did Richard. Already scolded by spirit, I lit the palo santo and rattled alongside Richard as he opened sacred space and called in the spirits of the four directions. He asked for the blessing of Pachamama, mother earth, thanking her for her sustenance, then Wirochocha, the great creator, for protection and wisdom, then east, south, west, and north, the condor, snake, jaguar and hummingbird. I could feel the presence of each animistic energetic presence, as he called them.

We then proceeded to say prayers and give kintus, florida water and tobacco as offerings to the spirits. I felt my heart open wide. As I journeyed into the spirit of the mountain I could feel my heart open. Emotional hurts, pains, and regrets came pouring out of my heart and were eaten up by the concentric rings of earth and stone. I flashed back to being ill with cancer and undergoing chemo and having people disassociate themselves from me, almost like they thought they would get cancer if they were near me. I also rarely saw my kids during that time of my life, as while I was so sick they had to live with their father. Pain seared though me as if it were physically tearing

Mystic Awakening of an AmericanPhysician
Linda Hostalek, D.O.

at my heart. I felt tears welling out of my eyes as I relived the pain of rejection from that time. I cried and cried and released that pain as my tears watered the ground below. Richard continue to rattle, and was also whistling, holding space for me to do this releasing work.

I realized through spirit, that just like I had tried to keep that beautiful rock that crumbled, sometimes things that look beautiful, like some friendships or relationships to people, things or ideas, can crumble in an instance if there is not a firm foundation. I realized that some people could not deal with my illness, and while it hurt me at the time, my heart now was becoming overwhelmed with release of this pain, and forgiveness of their desertion of me, which was really me releasing the expectation of people being there when I needed them, or thought I needed them. I realized that I was the one holding on to the pain, and felt great gratitude and appreciation for my life and for those who were there through the hard times. I relived the love and concern in my mother's eyes, and the fear in my children's. The pain left and was replaced with appreciation and joy. I even felt gratitude for those that hurt me, for I perceived no other way to learn this lesson of letting go and just loving all people and all things, for we are indeed one.

I felt the warm, loving embrace of Pachamama and her concentric circles of love. I came back to the consciousness of this reality with an overwhelming vulnerability. I was loved! I stood in the way of perceiving it and it cost me my happiness in the process. Had my love been tied to conditions? Well, that's not love, that's greed and manipulation, like me wanting the pretty, sparkly rock. Love is unconditional. I was loved unconditionally, and I needed to learn to love others unconditionally because that's the only kind of love there truly is. I looked at the crumbly, sparkly sand and held it in my hand. I thanked it for the lesson of the heart it just showed me. My tears were now of joy. I returned the rock that had become sand back to the earth, but kept a little to remind me of the healing beauty of this place. We closed space and just sat there for a while, quietly soaking up the energy.

Mystic Awakening of an AmericanPhysician
Linda Hostalek, D.O.

Richard held me in his arms and dried away my tears. "You are doing well," he told me. "It's not always easy to release the past, but it is necessary if you are to proceed and grow."

"I guess," I said quietly, feeling extremely vulnerable and yet strong at the same time. I was really glad to just 'be,' and it felt wonderful.

We began the ascent up the rings, feeling the temperature change, cooler with each successive ring, until we reached the top. I looked over the ringed landscape, how the three sets of rings merged with the mountain's natural contours, and again thanked the mountain for the very beautiful gift of healing. I looked down and spirit invited me to look closer. There laid a beautiful small stone, which contained some of those sparkles, but in a more stable rock form. I asked spirit's permission this time to pick it up and keep it. It said it was for me, a keepsake of my lesson here. I thankfully picked up the rock, and placed it in my mesa. My mesa was growing and my lessons were intense, but I was so thankful for this experience of being here, absorbing the beautiful energies.

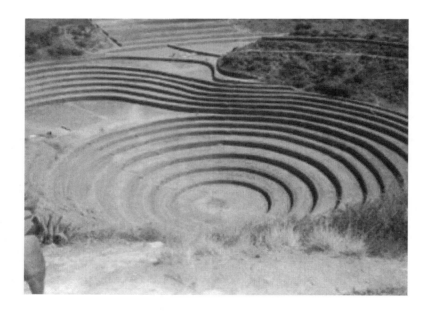

Chapter Eight

Where Heaven Lives

After breakfast, we had a driver take us to the lush
and magical site of Tipon. As we drove up the
winding road to the top of the mountain, I breathed in
the mountain air and the majestic sense of wonder
that only strong natural places can emanate. Snow
capped mountain in the background held the sense of
sacredness that permeates the region. "Apus," or
mountain angels, hold the space between the worlds,
of the heaven and the earth, where all life as we know
it exists. How holy it was to be in their presence. The
healing of yesterday in Moray was still on my mind,
and I felt less and less like a human, and more and
more like pure spirit. Vulnerable, quiet, sensitive, all

the vibrations of this place felt louder than normal. As we climbed to the sky, we arrived at Tipon. "We're here," Richard said. I got out of the car. The power of this place was amazing.

"What is this place?" I asked, a bit puzzled. I felt a heavenly presence penetrate this place; the 'I am', the all and the nothing. I was awed. I took my brown leather backpack, with my mesa and my water, and slung it over my shoulder. It was a bit cool, so I had a couple of layers on over my pink tank top and jeans. My hiking boots, a bit beat-up, seemed extra heavy that day.

Richard just smiled, like he had a secret he couldn't wait to show me. His skin, somewhat tan from the past few days, glowed a bit more than usual. He grabbed his satchel, with his mesa and accessories in it, paid the driver and arranged a pickup time.

"This is Tipon, the land of holy water, of the blending of the energies." He pointed to the distance, where we would hike to from here. "Here there is sacred water. It comes from a natural spring, and was

excavated by the ancients to create these sacred
channels." He smiled, like this was home for him. It
was easy to see he had been here many times
before.

I felt quiet and introverted that day. The sun came out
and as we hiked to the site, the layers came off. I
could feel the energies of this place, and we came
upon the lower channels. Water flowed from these
channels for hundreds of years, and as I crossed to
the other side I felt residual densities flowing away
from me as I passed over the running water. I
crossed over and back again, each time experiencing
the same thing. The emotional aspects of yesterday
seemed so far away, and today was a day of
cleansing. "I feel the cleansing of this water," I said
to Richard. "This is amazing!"

"This land is very holy," he said. "Here you have the
male aspect of spirit, the energy of the sun,
impregnating the land, and the female aspect of
Pachamama, the flowing of the water. These waters
come from holy underground springs, called
pakarinas, and are very special." He paused for a

moment, soaking up the energy, then began to walk again and said "Come here, I want to show you something."

He took me to a place where the water flowed over a hand hewn Incan cross, three quarters of the way up to where the water flowed in. The water landed in a squarish basin that forked off into two ribbons of flowing water flowing two ways. From a distance, it looked like a fully formed Incan cross, also called a chakana. Coming closer in, I felt the presence of the being of this magical place. I instinctively put my hands out to touch the water when Richard said, "Linda, come here, I want to show you the Incan spirit here." As I came to where he was he pointed to the fountain I was at and outlined a series of small outcroppings in the rock, "When the sun is right, it hits these markers, and the outline of the being is revealed, although I'm sure you can feel his presence here." He smiled a gigantic grin-- this is what he wanted to show me! It really was quite amazing. The Incan warrior holding his hands out to catch the water, just as I had done.

Mystic Awakening of an AmericanPhysician
Linda Hostalek, D.O.

I lingered at that area for a while, because I didn't want to leave it, but we were heading up to the top, where more sacred areas lay. As we hiked up the site, the sun warming us with its light, we came upon many sacred fountains. One turned into two, and two turned into four, each cascading down in a sacred dance of unity. Here male and female merged in balance. The vibration of this place was pure spirit. Balanced, it was neither male nor female; it was where one's soul could touch heaven, and mine did. We sat where we could see the fountains, and opened our mesas and began ceremony. My third eye began to open.

As my spirit merged with this holy place I was taken up to another realm. My body didn't matter, all densities were gone, and I was met by a being made of white light. Vaguely human-like, with a white bird head, I merged into one with this entity into the great one-ness of all life. Unimaginable beauty, peace, and joy merged with the bliss of appreciation for everything-- the air, the water, the mountains, the inter-connective-ness of all things, and my place in it.

Mystic Awakening of an AmericanPhysician

"This is where heaven lives," I thought to my self. "I never want to leave here."

Spirit began to show me how the ancients used this place to honor the creator god, Wiracocha. I saw despachos, fires, dances, and chants, but most of all I could see, feel, hear and taste the love-filled prayers of those that had gone before me. Sweet, beautiful and light, this was a a place of light, of thanksgiving and praise for the one who gives life. My consciousness was out of this clay body; I could see and feel the ancients Apus holding the worlds apart so that the frail race of humans could have a place to live. I also saw how little we appreciate it, and are generally ignorant of this. All I could say in this journey was, "Thank you, thank you, thank you!"

As the rattle brought me back down to earth and back in my body, I felt a whole new appreciation for my life, and the life of all on this earth. I looked up and saw a condor fly by. Spirit spoke loudly that day, to show me all that I and all peoples have to be thankful for. The holy beings that hold the cold vacuum of space from the fiery core of our earth, to make way for trees, soil,

Mystic Awakening of an AmericanPhysician
Linda Hostalek, D.O.

rocks, animals, plants, and humans. The trees and the atmosphere hold in place the holy cycle of water, which holds the keys for the life on this planet. This place was dedicated to all that is sacred. Thank you felt extremely inadequate for what I felt at that place.

"Its good, huh?" Richard smiled widely as he said, "This is one of my favorite places."

"Mine too. Thank you so much for bringing me here," I said as I smiled from deep inside my spirit, transformed once again by this magical, mystical land and this wonderful guide who came into my life to show me all this. I had waited for this my whole life, and here I was, experiencing my deepest desires, cleaning my soul and preparing my spirit. I felt relaxed, refreshed, rejuvenated and renewed. I just wanted to drink this in forever. I looked down and saw a lovely dark brown feather, a gift from the gods and this place. I treasured that wonderful gift, and added it to my ever growing mesa.

If Sasayhuman was the belly, and moray the heart, this had to be the head and spirit, the hannapacha.

Mystic Awakening of an AmericanPhysician

We headed back to Cuzco and drove down the
winding road in the presence of the holy Apus. My
transformation was now in full swing. We were on our
way to Machu Picchu, the ancient crystal city
tomorrow.

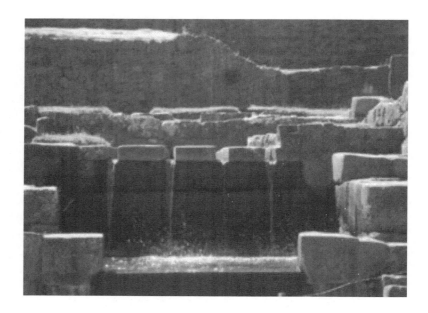

Chapter Nine

Machu Picchu

Morning came very early, but I was as excited as I could be. Today we were going to Machu Picchu - the lost crystal city! "Wake up sleepyhead!" Richard said as he handed me my clothes. I managed to get dressed quickly, and hurriedly packed a small bag as we were going to stay in the town of Agua Calientes, at the base of Machu Picchu.

We locked the rest of our belongings in a room at the hotel where we were staying, and departed for the train. We had some breakfast as we waited at the station, watching the people go by. There was a mixture of all types, young, old, families, travelers, speaking several languages. There was a cosmopolitan air to take in everywhere. We were on the vista view train, the most expensive ticket, due to the clear view. We boarded and took our seat, and away we went.

The view was amazing, like being swallowed by the mountains. Green, lush mountain tops gave way to more verdant mountains. Some had terraces and ruins on the side. Occasionally there would be a farmer with some llamas, but there was always the river. The Urubomba river guided us towards Agua Calientes. Rough and beautiful, large, rounded boulders encouraged white rapids to blast past anything in its way. She was strong and full of beauty, mystery and awe. I just stared out the window taking in the breathtaking scenery. "That's the river near where my blue-green rock came from!" I said, almost shocked, knowing so deep in my heart that was true.

"Very good," said Richard. "Your tracking skills are developing. You should be able to tell from any rock where it is from. When I was learning tracking, Jose Luis threw my cuellas, and I had to find them all. I did, but it wasn't easy," he laughed.

Mystic Awakening of an AmericanPhysician
Linda Hostalek, D.O.

Suddenly there was loud music, and a man dressed
in a white outfit with a full face mask with colored eyes
and mouth, came out from the front of the train car.
He had a cape, and he danced a magical dance with
a bit of darkness to it, but very powerful. This was the
devil character from a festival somewhat like Carnival,
both disturbing and provocative. Then there was a
fashion show of high end alpaca products, very
beautiful and expensive, and oh so soft. We were
then offered a meal, and continued our ride.

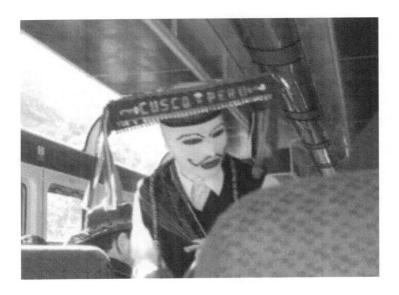

Mystic Awakening of an AmericanPhysician

As we got closer to Agua Calientes, the entire vibe changed. The trees got more tropical, the air had more humidity, and the vibration of silent drums stirred in my heart. "We're getting close," he whispered to me, as I smiled with my head on his shoulder, still staring at the mountain view above and the dangerously wild river below.

"This is amazing," was all I could say. I had experienced more in the past few days than many people experience in a lifetime it seemed, and I just tried to take it all in. The time in Cuzco clearing my belly, in Moray healing my heart, and Tipon healing my soul-- I couldn't even begin to imagine what would take place here in Machu Picchu. I silently thanked the mountains and river as we passed by, and then we were finally coming to the end of our line.

"We're here, so grab your bag, and hold on to it. Sometimes people try to grab things off tourists," he said as he pulled me towards him so I wouldn't get lost in the crowd. He held my hand and after we passed through the crowded exit lane, we passed into Agua Calientes.

Mystic Awakening of an AmericanPhysician
Linda Hostalek, D.O.

It was much warmer than Cuzco, and the air felt more tropical. I noticed I could breathe easier and took a big, deep breath. Richard looked at me and said, "Easier to breathe, huh?"

"Much easier!" It felt good to breathe deeply again, and I hadn't realized just how compromised my breathing had been.

"It's a lot lower elevation here, but it's pretty high up there...." Richard turned and pointed skywards towards the very large mountain top. "Just over that ridge is where we will be going tomorrow. All the buses have already left for the day, so let's go find a place to stay. I want to look up a couple of people I know."

Agua Calientes was a small town that existed mostly to serve the few tourists who made the effort to get there. There were a few shops set up in a make-shift market, selling some crystals, jewelry, and other tourist tokens, but there was little to pick from and the town shut down pretty early. It was probably about 3 or 4 o'clock in the afternoon, and people were already shutting down their kiosks, as ours was the last train.

There were a few restaurants across an old wooden bridge, and a lot of construction seemed to be going on, although I saw no workers.   The train tracks ended on a board walk with large wooden sidewalks and some restaurants. They were all closed. We walked across to the center of town a couple of blocks away. There was a main square plaza with a few open restaurants where the locals were gathered having some drinks and food. Several small cobblestone side-streets radiated out from the square, and Richard took my hand and said, "Let's go this way," and we passed by what looked to be houses, then found one that had a small sign that said 'vacancy.' We went and found our home for the next few days.

Our room was on the second floor overlooking some treetops and the neighbors' rooftop. There were cactus drying on the roof, several slices to the plate. "What is that?" I asked. "Why are they drying it on the roof?"

Mystic Awakening of an AmericanPhysician
Linda Hostalek, D.O.

"Oh, that is San Pedro. It is a hallucinogenic plant medicine that produces great visions. They harvest the cactus, dry it in the sun, then brew it in to the medicine when it is ready. It takes a long time to do the entire process." Richard explained.

"Will we be taking that medicine?" I asked.

"No, not this time. Perhaps at a different time. You need to be at a different level in your training. Some people take it and do not respect the plant spirit behind it. It is very powerful medicine." He said sternly. "You will be ready soon, but always remember to respect the plant and its teachings."

"What does it do?" I asked.

"It depend on the intent of the user, and of the plant. The plant spirit is alive, and when respected, can be a most wonderful teacher. There is also a jungle plant, a vine, called auyahauscha, or the vine of the dead. Both help one to cross over to the other side."

Mystic Awakening of an AmericanPhysician

"Really?" I asked, intrigued with the idea of what was on the other side.

"Really," he said, and pulled me to him and we christened the new room with our passionate lovemaking. I felt like I was falling in love. I just wasn't sure with what. Was it Richard? The entire experience of other worldly realms? This place was so beautiful. I began to wonder how he felt about me. Was he falling in love with me too? It felt that way. I tried to put those thoughts out of my mind and we headed out to dinner.

We walked hand in hand down the cobblestone street. Lined with small outdoor eateries, and a few shops, we stopped at a place that was still partially under construction. "What are we doing here?" I asked.

"Oh, my friend Machu Picchu Bob lives here now."

"Is he Peruvian?" I asked.

"No, he's American," Richard said with a grin on his face.

Mystic Awakening of an AmericanPhysician
Linda Hostalek, D.O.

"Why is he called Machu Picchu Bob?"

"A couple of years ago, I was leading a group here," he looked reflectively towards the mountains' direction, a wry smile crossed his face, "and we had just done ceremony on the top where the Intihuantana, the hitching post of the sun is. Well, Bob, who had always been a very rational man, heard the voice of spirit talking to him, and it said to jump off the cliff!"

"Jump off the cliff?!" I said, startled that that could happen. "What happened then? I mean, he couldn't have jumped.."

"Yeah, he did!" Richard interrupted. "He heard Spirit's voice tell him to jump and that he would be okay, and then he had to stay. And so-- he jumped! Right off the side of the mountain!"

"You're kidding, right?" I said, half not believing.

"No, its true. He landed in a pile of brush on the side of the mountain, we needed to get a helicopter to air-lift him out of the pile, and then they took him to the hospital."

"Was he badly hurt?" I wondered.

"No, just some bumps and bruises. He had to pay a big fee though. Helicopters aren't cheap!" He laughed. "Now he lives here." We approached the small stone and adobe like structure and Richard knocked on the door. A medium built, white man, about 50, with long gray hair, and a long gray beard came to meet us.

"Richard!" The man said, obviously very happy to see him. "Hi, I'm Bob," he said to me, and invited us in. He was turning this place into a healing center with massage and energy healing. "Here will be the massage room," Bob said as he led us into a half finished room with stone tiles on the floor, and stained glass in the window. "Here will be the kitchen," and so on throughout the structure. He radiated happiness and peace. I would come to find out after

Mystic Awakening of an AmericanPhysician
Linda Hostalek, D.O.

the helicopter incident, he sold his house, quit his lucrative job as a stockbroker, and moved to Agua Calientes to give his service to spirit. He had met a local woman and the two of them would be running this place as soon as it was finished.

We invited them to come share a meal with us, but they were unable to do so, so we went on further up the road towards the hot baths. The name Agua Caliente means 'hot water' and the region is known for its geothermal springs. We had a nice light dinner, the headed further up towards the baths. We passed the place where construction ended, and just the road continued. We came upon a small rock shop, and we felt compelled to check it out. This place felt spiritual, and we looked at the rocks and jewelry in the window and decided we would come back later when it was open.

We continued on to edge of town where the baths were. We changed in to our suits and immersed ourselves in the hot, healing waters. Any aching muscles immediately were soothed, and any lingering stress melted. I felt heavenly. In love with life, maybe with Richard, and more than a bit tired. I began to wonder again how he felt.

We finished our bath and began the walk home. The moon was out and full, and the scent of tropical flowers filled the air with perfume. I don't know what made me feel I needed to know right then and there, but I did. "Richard?" I asked, "Do you love me?" I felt foolish, but I just wanted an answer. I'm here, in a foreign country, experiencing amazing stuff, and although this is all new to me, I was aware that this was not new to him.

"Of course I love you," he said. "I created you, how could I not love you?"

Now I was a bit confused. What did that mean? Did that mean I created him too? I decided to just let it go at that. I was tired, overtired, and perhaps just a little bit whiney. We walked back to our room and made love again. He made it a point to tell me "I love you" frequently after that. I guess I needed to hear that. My insecurities were beginning to pop up. I felt better, and I slept with a peace in my heart. Clean, clear, and very tired, I fell into a deep slumber.

Mystic Awakening of an American Physician
Linda Hostalek, D.O.

We woke up, we made love and off we went to the
bus station that would take us up the great mountain.
Today would be one of the most important days of my
life, although I had no idea just how important then.
We waited for the bus. It took a while to get there.
Back in those days, they ran few and far between, not
on the schedule that they have now. We climbed in
and began the adventure.

First we drove past where the train-tracks ended.
There was a beautiful new hotel under construction
there, workers taking a break on the street. Past a
bridge and a footpath, then the ascent began. The
bus climbed up the steep slope of the mountain back
and forth, with very sharp turns. Midway between
turns, where the relatively straight part was, a
waterfall diverted water from the road to the tunnel
below. Once another bus came and we had to share
the road to allow them to pass, I could hardly believe
we were still on the mountain after pulling off so far to
the side. Nerve-wracking if I looked down, I tried to
keep my eyes on the mountains facing us. "There is
Winay Picchu. This is Machu Picchu." Richard began

to name all the mountains, distracting me from the dangerous curves our bus was navigating. We passed through the mist and arrived at our destination at the top of the mountain. Relieved and excited, we got out.

This was like nothing else! I looked over to the mountain across. Birds soared on the thermals below us, and mist from clouds floated beneath us. "Pretty amazing, huh?" Richard said. "This is one of my favorite places."

"I can see why. I have always wanted to come here, I can hardly believe I'm here!" I said, as I squeezed his hand. We gave our tickets to the guard at the booth, and entered the ancient ground that spoke with the whispers of the ancestors. We toured the lower part of the complex first. He showed me the curved windows where the sun would hit at sunrise on the equinoxes and solstices. We then moved to the natural cave with the condor carved into the stone on the floor, and he invited me to feel the energy of this magical place. We crossed ancient runnels and fountains with holy water flowing. He cleansed his energy body with the water, and invited me to do the same. Just like we did in Tipon, I held the water in my cupped hands and splashed it onto my belly, heart, and forehead to clean my three centers. It was very refreshing, and I could hear echoes of the spirits welcoming me to this sacred land.

After a while, we passed the long grassy area and began to ascend to where the holy of holies was, the Intihuantana, the hitching post of the sun. We were by the quarry, near the sacred area, when Richard announced, "I need to go visit an area over there." He pointed to the far section of the complex, "I'll be back in a while, I'll find you, go explore here and see what you find."

Before I could speak, he was gone. I lost it. All forms of feelings came into my body; anger, rage, abandonment, fear, foolishness, all came surging through my body like a lightning bolt. I could feel fire-like energy coming out of my feet through my boots. Pain in my upper right abdomen kept feeling like fire exiting through my boots! I stomped and kicked and cried like a child. I wanted to run away, since I felt so foolish. I saw some steps that led to the top of an adjoining mountain. I flew up those steps due to the fire jet engine propulsion coming out of my boots! I flew up that mountain. I ran so fast and with each step felt more and more toxic anger come out my feet. Years of pain of abandonment, feelings of failure, not being loved, and conditional love flew out my feet. I felt ashamed, embarrassed, and foolish.

When I reached the top of the mountain I was afraid if I went any further I would get lost and not be able to find my way back. I sat down on the rock and cried and cried and cried. I couldn't help myself. Years of anger, disguised in so many forms, melted out of me. With each sob, the tears were cleansing, healing, and eventually brought me strength and peace. I heard a hum near my left ear. As I lifted my head off my folded arms, I saw a beautiful hummingbird, iridescent, with two very long tail feathers less than a foot away from my face, feeding on a yellow flower. I turned and looked at the landscape I just ran from; I could see the entire complex of Machu Picchu. Magnificent! The power of that moment is etched in my memory forever.

Mystic Awakening of an AmericanPhysician
Linda Hostalek, D.O.

I realized that all those memories were instances
where I had given away my power, not asserted my
self, or otherwise would not let myself engage in
anger. I had repressed my anger and it came out full
steam!   But it felt good, liberating, free; I was
released from the bondage of my own anger! I made
friends with my anger that day-- to this day that is one
of the most helpful things I have ever learned. I
realized that anger serves a purpose-- to warn us
when something is not right. Far too often I had
repressed that anger in the moment, stuffing it down
inside, where it could fester into depression, or even
cancer. Anger sets up a disturbing pattern that if not
dealt with effectively, can wreck havok on one's
energy system, like it did on mine.

That is why I had been so clingy. After being
cleansed and refreshed on one level with the visits to
the sacred sites, the underlying insecurities could
come to the surface. No one, not even Richard, could
help me understand why I felt like that; I had to
experience it for myself. That is why I needed to have
this experience, and I really 'got it.' The hummingbird

showed me that life is incredible, including the dramas that as a human, I had created to teach myself these lessons of life. I was God-smacked once again-- cracking my spirit open like a parrot does to nuts!

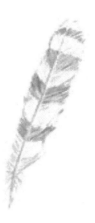

I caught my breath and took in the beauty of this moment. After I stopped crying, the hummingbird quietly left. I intuited that it was there to show me the magic in all things great and small. The wild, majestic mountains, the fragile mountain flower, the incredible hummingbird, all converging to show me how to transform and no longer be bound by my own demons. That was all there is, demons we create ourself, in my case, abandonment issues. That was MY issue, not others'. We only live in this brief second before another passes and that one is gone forever. I learned that to be happy is to stay in the moment, not the future or the past, but the now! I am eternally grateful to the spirit of the hummingbird.

I looked around and noticed that where I was perched was the end of the Inca trail, the hike that some adventurous souls travel on for several days, and their reward is the vision I was now beholding. It was a living postcard. I was again refreshed, renewed and rejuvenated. Richard knew I needed to finish my healing process on my own. I was so grateful to him for leaving me to experience this awesome experience which would not have been possible any other way.

I began making my way down the rocky steps that I so easily flew up. As I came down further back into Machu Picchu proper, I noticed a small natural cave in the side of the mountain. I crawled in, and began ceremony. It hadn't even occurred to me then that this was the first time I ever did ceremony on my own.

Mystic Awakening of an AmericanPhysician

I opened my mesa, spritzed florida water, rattled and opened sacred space. I made kintus and thanked Pachamama for the beauty, wonder and transformation of this holy place, and Wirococha for holding me safely throughout it all. The cave was alive, and on a small ledge, I noticed a cubby hole, and a chubby, furry creature came out to meet me, followed by another. They looked kind of like rabbits, but the ears were smaller, and the tails were long. They were grayish brown, and very furry. They were happy to meet me, to welcome me here, and they were pleased with my presence. I was filled to the brim with appreciation. I had come full circle. I thanked those beings, who I would find out much later were chinchillas, or andean rabbits, and left the cave to find Richard. To this day, that cave holds a very special place in my heart, and years later I would return to this cave with my own apprentice, but that, too, is a story for a different time.

Mystic Awakening of an AmericanPhysician
Linda Hostalek, D.O.

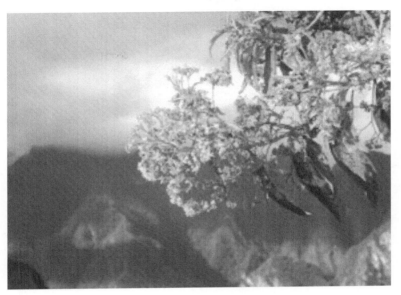

Mystic Awakening of an AmericanPhysician

Chapter Ten

Initiation

Refreshed from making friends with my anger and talking with the hummingbird and chinchillas, I made my way to the base of the sacred site. Richard was there waiting for me. He gave me that knowing look and nodded his head. "You are ready," he said. I felt that I was, and he could see that I was changed.

We walked to the top of the mountain, just outside where the Intihuatana, the hitching post of the sun, was enclosed with stone ruins. This area had a room with three windows, for watching the summer and winter solstices, and the equinoxes. Just outside this area, in the plaza area near the stairs to the

Mystic Awakening of an AmericanPhysician

Intihuantana, was a very large, grey stone. Flat, with a slight angle, it looked like a giant stone bed. At least 20 inches tall, it was about 5 or 6 feet wide and about 8 feet long. Richard told me "That is the death stone. Years ago, shamans would get their initiation rites on this mountain," he motioned to the space past the doorway where the Intihuatana was. "The master shaman would call in the spirits while the initiate would see if they were accepted by the spirits as they lay on this stone. If accepted, they would then proceed to the Intihuantana."

This was a heady place, since the spirit of the ancestors was very strong here. As I looked out past the three windows, the green misty foliage of the adjacent mountain glowed ephemerally. On the other side, the vast blue sky separated the next mountain as a condor flew on the thermals. I was speechless.

"Lay down here," Richard instructed as he motioned me to lay on the death stone.

"OK," I said, somewhat trembling as to what would happen next, but ready.

Mystic Awakening of an AmericanPhysician
Linda Hostalek, D.O.

Now he got serious. His eyes flashed with a brilliance
that transcended time and space. His face morphed
into that of an ancestor as he began to rattle and go
into a trance. I soon found myself also in a trance,
and as I lay down, my mesa on my belly, I found
myself floating into an alternate reality. I floated out of
my body and merged with the sky. I could see and
feel every star in space; the southern cross, the eyes
of the llama, were in my soul.

Condors, jaguars, and serpents danced in my spirit,
while hummingbirds danced me to the outer limits of
the galaxies; from the ether of space, I felt two
etheric arms holding me and cradling me. These
were the arms of Apu Machu Picchu holding me! I
belonged here. It felt so right. Bathed in luminous
layers of colors, light and love, I turned into a
hummingbird and soared in the sky. Wirococha lifted
me, and at the same time Pachamama held me.

Everywhere and nowhere at the same time, I now
understood the week's previous healings. I needed to
be purified to be here at his level, and to make friends

with my anger to make way for love, light and healing. The spirits had accepted me, the honor of that moment brought tears to my eyes. My spirit came back into my body, and I came back to this reality. I opened my eyes, and now noticed that there were others around me, tourists, who were watching this special event. I sat up, and sat on that stone for a while.

"Now you are ready," Richard said. I could see the father-like pride in his eye. I think I even saw a hint of a tear. He held out his hand and took mine to lift me off the stone. We walked up the nearby stairs to the place where the crown jewel was, the Intihuantana, a huanka, or place where the spirit impregnates the earth, usually intepreted as a male phallus symbol. The Intihuantana at Machu Picchu is one of the most important huankas in all of Peru.

Intihuantana was also called 'The hitching post of the sun.' It was called that because the sun is held in place, or hitched, there during the two equinoxes of the year in March and September. Cut from the highest peak of this holy mountain, it was the most sacred site here. Legend said that to touch the forehead to the Intihuantana would open the third eye. The Spanish destroyed other huankas, in an attempt to destroy the Inca culture, but they never discovered Machu Picchu, so its Intihuantana remained intact. An aura of energy was visibly pouring out it at every angle. The base was larger than the Intihuatana itself, making it even more impressive as it rose into the sky. On one side were steps leading up to the sacred huanka. "Here is where you walk, to give your prayers to the sun, for thanksgiving, and for blessing," Richard said. "Are you ready?"

"Yes, I am ready. Thank you," I said, and I silently went to the side, bent my head, held my mesa close, and ascended up the steep, narrow steps to the side of the Intihuatana, wind blowing through my hair. I said my prayers of thanksgiving silently with each mindful step, then aloud when I reached the top, finding a song in my heart that needed to be sung in praise, right then, right there. I placed a kintu on the base near the upward portion of the Intihuatana, kneeled in front of it, and placed my forehead over the rope and on to the Intihuatana. It was finished. This was where God lived, and it was the most beautiful place I had ever seen. Now I understood why Machu Picchu Bob jumped, and why it took a helicopter to get him down! I merged a piece of my soul with that place that day, and it has stayed with me ever since. The hitching post of the Sun, the place where God lives, was holding me, merging with me, and I would never be the same.

We lingered there a while, Richard pointing out that the rocks were in the same shapes as the mountains they represented in the background. This entire place was magical. We eventually made our way down to the more level area, where there is a large beautiful stretch of lawn. Several llamas would stop and graze in between walking around. These llamas and alpacas are considered sacred. A staple of the Quechua people, who used every part of these animals. Their wool was used for weavings and textiles, and they ate them on occasion. Even their fetuses, which would naturally abort frequently, would sometimes be used in their magical rituals. Some called them Andean camels, as they are related to their brothers and sisters on the other side of the world, for example, in Egypt, where they too are a decorated and celebrated part of their culture.

It had been a very full day. We sat on the lawn by the lone tree overlooking the mountain vista and stone structures. We opened our mesas and rattled to connect once more on this sacred site and to offer our prayers of thanksgiving. Again, my spirit flew and again I was one with the mountain. Machu Picchu was my spirit mountain, it had adopted me! Those same hands that had held me previously now held a white and silver braided band, with a single, erect, large, white feather, and placed it over my head energetically. I was an Inca Princess. I was told by Spirit that this is a temporary crown, almost like a training crown, and that when I was ready and had matured in this tradition, I would be receive a full crown.

Now I knew why I dreamt of this place my whole life and had always wanted to come here; why spirit made it so easy for me to get here when the time was right, and why the healings here were so intense for me. I was home, and no matter where I would ever venture, the energy of this place would, from here on out, always be living in my heart.

We walked out through the gates that separated the park from the entrance on the mountain. There was a small restaurant in the sky, and we were both a bit hungry after such a long day. "Are you hungry?" Richard asked me.

"Yes, a little," I said, although food didn't really seem all that important at that time.

"Let's get something here," he suggested.

I was in no hurry, so I said "OK."

We got some chips and salsa to eat and a couple of lemonades and went to sit at a table near the edge of the mountain side. The restaurant was built into the side of the mountain, and the patio with the table and chairs had a fence to keep you safe while you dined and overlooked the neighboring mountains. As I was taking a drink of my lemonade, I looked up at the mountain restaurant decor-- three spirals -- just like

Mystic Awakening of an AmericanPhysician
Linda Hostalek, D.O.

Richard placed in my energy field during the dream when he made love to me and penetrated the knowledge into me. Once again, confirmation from spirit that I was meant to be here and have this experience.

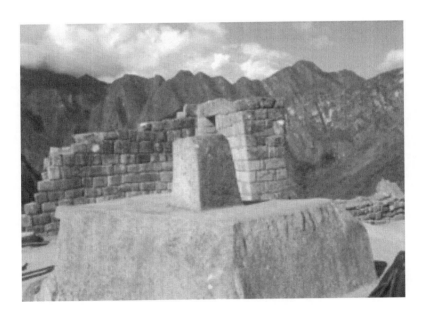

Mystic Awakening of an AmericanPhysician

Chapter Eleven

Afterglow

We took the long, winding bus back down to Agua
Calientes, went back to our room, made love, took a
shower, got dressed and went out for a real dinner.
The air was sweet and fresh as we walked hand in
hand through the square. We went down the same
cobbled street as we did the night before to get to the
baths, and looked for a place to have a proper meal.
We found a nice little place with blue and white tiled
floors, dark wooden doors and windows, white cloth
napkins, real silver utensils, and heavy white plates
and crystal glasses.

Mystic Awakening of an AmericanPhysician

Richard ordered us two piso sours, as we looked over the dinner menu. I didn't drink much, but this was a special occasion, and the piso sour is the official drink of the Andes. Piso is a heavy wine, sort of like a brandy, and when made into a sour, is made with lemon juice, sugar and egg whites whipped into a peak. It came out with a frothy white peak on top of lemony yellow liquid. It was quite good-- and very strong. I could only sip it slowly as I could feel each sip's warmth melt into a delicious orgy in my mouth.

I ordered some alpaca and Richard ordered a guinea pig, called coy. Both quite typical Peruvian dishes, both with pappas fritas, fried peruvian potatoes, of which Peru boasts several varieties. We laughed and celebrated our magical day, as well as the wonderful week. The alpaca tasted a lot like beef, and the guinea pig was a bit greasy for my taste, like a red meat chicken. We finished our delicious meal, and decided to take a little stroll around the town.

We walked to the town square, which was very typical of any Latin American city. Open air restaurants, a church, a fountain, some benches, music playing in the background, and smells of roasted meats continued the theme of deliciousness that night. As we were walking through the square, enjoying our evening, I noticed that something caught Richard's eye in a very intense way, and he turned and shouted "Jose Luis!"

"Ricardo?" said a voice. A warm smile spread across Richard's face as we made our way towards this man I had only heard about. "Come, sit!" There, on the square, sitting by himself on a small wooden bench near a table with a checkered tablecloth, in an open-air restaurant, was a man enjoying a beer, apparently waiting for some food.

This was the infamous Jose Luis. This was the man who grew up at the base of Machu Picchu and apprenticed under the revered Don Manuel Quispe. Jose Luis was Richard's mentor, friend, and teacher. He wore a dark purple expedition-type shirt and jacket, blue jeans and hiking boots. A handsome man, relatively tall, with dark curly hair that was not too short, and dark mysterious eyes, he had a friendly, humble demeanor, which belied his deep sensuality and love of life. His energy field was luminous.

It was obvious to me that this was a man who resonated deeply with spirit. I had heard tales of him bringing people back from being nearly dead, and how he could summon spirits-- and of his willingness to teach those that truly wanted, and were ready-- to walk the medicine path. Richard had been studying with him for several years already, and they had made many expeditions to holy mountains together. He would also teach in tandem with Richard in certain areas in the midwest.

We exchanged the usual pleasantries and introductions. Jose Luis ordered two more beers, one for Richard, one for me, and I sat down, mesmerized, as I could hardly believe I was in the presence of this man.

"Have you been with the others of the mission trip?" Richard asked, curious if they were back yet. He had not expected to see Jose Luis this evening.

Mystic Awakening of an AmericanPhysician
Linda Hostalek, D.O.

"No, I was with some others on a pilgrimage to Ausangante," Jose Luis said. "You would have enjoyed it, Ricardo, wonderful despachos and ceremony, just beautiful."

"We've had a bit of that ourselves this week." Richard informed him. "We went to Sachayhuman, Moray, and Tipon before we came here, and today, Linda got her initiation rites on the death stone at Machu Picchu."

Jose Luis looked at me, or rather right through me, and nodded, approvingly. "Very good," he said. "So, how do you feel?" he asked me, as I could feel his penetrating gaze scanning my energy field.

"I feel wonderful!" I told him, and related my story of my journey in as few words as I could. "Richard has told me a lot about you," I said, as I took another drink of my beer.

"You have learned a lot this week," Jose Luis said. "You have done well." I still don't know if that was for me or for Richard, but I was happy and it didn't matter. "Perhaps you can come by the hotel Cuzco tomorrow night, that's when the group will be back. I'm sure Holly and Michael would be happy to see you. They can tell you how the mission went."

"We heard there were rains," Richard said.

"There were, but they got a good start on them, so they should have been okay."

"We were supposed to go with them, but they said they had to leave early. We decided to come down anyway. It worked out well, I wouldn't have been able to take Linda to all those sacred sites and do ceremony otherwise."

Jose Luis looked right through me again, reading my energy. Again he smiled and nodded his head, and then he and Richard began to catch up-- two old friends catching up to the present since last they met.

We laughed and drank, and they smoked cigars. I felt like I just joined an exclusive club and I was its newest member, accepted, but still so much to learn.

Mystic Awakening of an AmericanPhysician
Linda Hostalek, D.O.

I felt so honored to be in the presence of these two men, sent to me by sprit, for lessons in life I could not yet comprehend.

Richard and I went back to our room, it was such an intense day and night. Richard was very excited to see Jose Luis, as was I. He took some special cigars out of his backpack and went back to the restaurant. I stayed in quiet contemplation of the past day's and week's events. I could feel we were getting ready to land in reality, and I wasn't ready to go yet. I would go tomorrow, while tonight I would enjoy the afterglow.

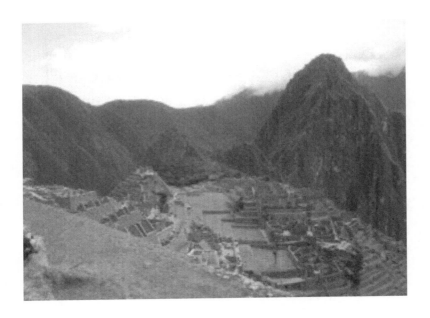

Mystic Awakening of an AmericanPhysician

Chapter Twelve

The Beginning of Reality

I woke up the next morning to misty rain tapping on the windowpanes. I got up to close the window, and noticed the medicinal cacti that were previously drying on the adjacent roof were gone, and a few bowls and pots were there instead, catching water in a melodious tinkling, like the rain itself was singing. I just sat there for a few moments, drinking in this view, and the way I felt. We would be leaving here this morning, and going back to Cuzco, and on to Lima the next day. This magical adventure was coming to an end, and going on to a new beginning. I snuck back in bed and woke Richard up. We savored that delicious morning; we both knew our time was limited here and so we made the most of it.

Mystic Awakening of an AmericanPhysician

After a lazy morning rendezvous, we finished packing our bags, and made our way to the train. Jose Luis had left the night before by car with a friend. He had a place in Cuzco, and he and Richard had planned to meet up with the rest of the group we missed earlier. They were staying in a Cuzco hotel, and there was going to be a farewell dinner that night before the Americans left for the states.

We took the regular train back to Cuzco. I remember that the mountains had spirit faces everywhere, and the outlines of those holy mountains looked like jaguars, serpents, and sensuous human forms. Creation, procreation, the health of the village's land and crops; these were important themes. Spirit was everywhere, and I knew that I could understand that it was everywhere better, if only I took the time to look. I remembered the different patients, who showed me spiritual and emotional imbalances that reflected in their chakras and bodies, were very similar to the reverence, health and vibrancy, or lack of them, in the land. My own land at home needed some of this healing reverence; I began thinking of ways to improve things there.

Home was calling me back. I realized I didn't dwell on my home while I had been away. I had been totally immersed in this transformation, and now my lessons needed to be brought back home. I was watching the outlines of the mountains out the train window, when Richard leaned over, put his arm around me, and said, "Thoughts?"

"I was just thinking about home. This place is so special, and it will live in my heart forever, and I was wondering, how do I bring this feeling home?" I asked, as I snuggled up closer.

"You are linked forever to this place now. Anytime you want, you can connect here by going into sacred space and calling on the holy Apus," he hugged me tight and said "Don't worry, this feeling won't go away."

"Don't you think things will be different when we get back?"

Mystic Awakening of an AmericanPhysician

"Just like you can feel home here, you will be able to feel here back home," Richard said reassuringly. "The invisible energetic lines that link you to home, or to here, are called cekes. They are like invisible light strings, and you can choose where to be linked." His eyes smiled with warmth, "Besides, you still have training to do, and I'm not going away."

I smiled at that thought.

We finally arrived in Cuzco and made our way back to our hotel where we had stayed previously. We took our stuff out of storage, took a shower and changed our clothes. We were to meet the group at a different hotel, and from there we were going to go to one of the shamans' houses for a celebration feast.

We arrived at a nice hotel, with several people waiting in the lobby. Most were dressed in clean hiking type clothes and hiking boots, some in jeans, and two ladies were wearing flowing dresses, made of gauze-like material. The group looked tired, like they just got off the mountain, which they did earlier that afternoon.

Mystic Awakening of an AmericanPhysician
Linda Hostalek, D.O.

They looked happy to see Richard, and he began to introduce me to all his friends.

One of the people he knew was a little Peruvian woman, probably about fifty, with steely black eyes, and her black hair pulled back in double braids. Her name was Dona Bernadina, and her black, gauzy dress was emblazoned with bright colorful flowers. She wore a matching head covering, as a sign of respect to the spirits. She was a priestess, and a masterful healer, I would come to find out in later years. She had a spritely look that made her look much younger than she really was. "How was the trip?" Richard asked.

"Very muddy," she said in her broken English, smiling. "A few of the horses slipped, but everyone made it up to the top okay. You come to my house tonight-- okay, we made you coy, you like the coy, yes?" You could see she was very excited to have all these people come to her house.

We piled into four different cars, and drove a little out of town. We pulled up to a large, metal, utilitarian gate, amid a whole block of cement block fences. There were a few cars on the streets, but it mostly looked dark and unoccupied. One of the men got out and opened the gate, and all the cars pulled inside.

Inside was a cement parking pad, and a very large garden area, like a buffer zone between the street and the house. There was a small, well-maintained, stucco, one-story home up the walkway. Flowers of every color exploded out of a myriad of containers, planters, and the ground itself. It smelled like heaven. There was a building about the size of a garage, that had two long, hand-hewn tables and some wooden chairs and benches. It was also made of white stucco, and it had no windows. Other than six large, hand-painted, oil portraits of spiritual beings hung on the walls, there was no other decoration.

I would come to learn that this was a gathering place for the shamans, a church of sorts, for calling spirit, making despachos and doing ceremony. The portraits were painted by this lady's son, himself an apprentice shaman, who had seen those spirits, those angelic messengers, in his ceremonies.

Mystic Awakening of an American Physician
Linda Hostalek, D.O.

Dona Bernadina brought out platters of meat, bowls of
salad, and dishes of grains. Jose Luis and Dona
Bernadina thanked spirit for and blessed the food,
and we sat down and ate. There was coy, the guinea
pig fried golden brown, roasted chicken, multiple side
dishes, desserts, coffee, and soft drinks. We ate,
drank, and listened to tales of the last week's events.
I was really glad things worked out the way they did.
It sounded like an arduous trip up the mountain, and I
wouldn't have missed the past week Richard and I
had for anything. It did sound ideal though, trekking
up the mountain, taking care of the local kids, bringing
them gifts, and living in their community for that time.

"The school is coming along nicely," said Holly, one of
the Americans who was a mission veteran. "You
should see how big little Maria is, she's probably
grown six inches!" She had a brown shirt and cargo
pants, short brown hair, and a big grin with a small
gap between her two front teeth. A bit stocky, she
held her energy like she was a few inches taller than
her five foot, three inch frame. She and Richard had

been friends for many years, going on these trips for several years now.

"How is Freida? Did she have her baby yet?" Richard asked.

"No, but it shouldn't be long; we did a despacho for her and the baby," Holly continued, "It was a nice time after the rough start," she said, sounding rather matter-of-fact.

They were busy talking about all kinds of events and people they knew, and I went to speak to Jose Luis. He invited me to sit by him, and he then asked me, "So, how did you meet Richard?"

I told him the longer version of the story I told him the night before, then I asked, "Do you come to the states often?"

"Oh, yes," he laughed. "I have a place where I stay in Virginia. I have a brother who lives there. I used to live in St. Louis, where I studied civil engineering." He reached over to get another piece of chicken, "Now I teach this medicine path. Richard is one of my apprentices who did his work, and now he teaches as well. Sometimes we teach together."

"Do you have any plans to come to the states and teach anytime soon?" I asked.

"Well, Richard and I have a weekend planned for June, near Wisconsin, around the solstice, you may want to come to that." Jose Luis said, as he smiled wide. "I have a feeling you will be around."

"I would love that!" I said. "I'll talk to Richard and make the arrangements."

"Wonderful!" he said, and I could tell by his energy that he really meant it.

I met many wonderful people that night, and all too quickly it was time to leave. We piled into the cars, and drove back into Cuzco near the city square. Richard and I were dropped off first, while the others were driven back to their hotel. With the passion of two lovers who would not see each other for an undetermined time, we made the most of our time together.

Mystic Awakening of an AmericanPhysician

Morning came very early the next day. We gathered our belongings and the driver loaded our bags in the taxi and drove us to the Cuzco airport. I said goodbye to this magical land, and vowed that I would be back someday. After an uneventful flight to Lima, we discovered we had a very long layover, so we checked our international bags, put our carry-ons into a locker, and took a taxi to the Gold Museum.

We saw many ancient treasures there, skulls made of crystals, human skulls with teeth replaced with gems, many pieces of jewelry, like bracelets, rings, and earrings, laid next to breastplates made of gold, and many other artifacts. The energy in that place was very strong, as if voices from the afterlife demanded recognition even in death. Next to the Gold Museum was a display of textiles from all over Peru. The weavings were colorful, with many similar themes, such as the chakana, or Incan cross, or that mountain type of x that I saw in Cuzco and was woven into my mesa cloth. There were also prints from the jungle. Those were more psychedelic in nature, with bright

186

blues and reds, reflecting their cosmology. They were all beautiful.

We went to the seaside afterwards, and had our last meal in Peru. We dined on cerviche, a pickled white fish with peppers and onions, marinated in lime juice, which actually 'cooks' the fish with its acidity. We got to view the Pacific ocean before we needed to go back to the airport to catch our midnight flight.

We got back to the airport, through security (pre 9/11), and found our way to our gate. To our surprise, a few of the Americans from the mission group were also waiting for their plane there as well. They left on an earlier flight than us, but it was still nice to spend some time with them again. It was time to return to reality, but we all knew we would be back. Pachamama lived in my soul, because I was now a part of this land. With a knowingness that this would somehow be integrated into my life on all levels, I wondered exactly how this would affect my life once I got home.

Mystic Awakening of an AmericanPhysician

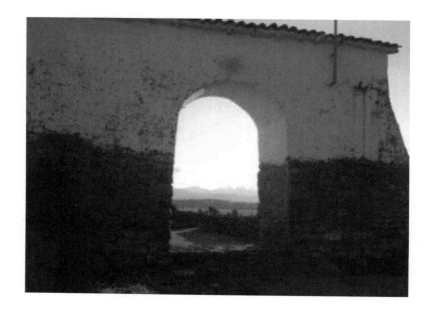

Chapter Thirteen

The End is the Beginning

I returned home to my boys and my condo with different eyes. Everything was a gift from God. I began my 'official' shaman training with Richard and Jose Luis a couple months after we returned. Richard and I continued our relationship for a while, but after a period of wonderful transformations with the plant medicines, it was time to move on for both of us. I continued to study with Jose Luis for the next decade plus, eventually training my own apprentices and bringing them on their own journey to the magical land that claimed my heart. My western medicine also blossomed, as spirit would continue to show me the relationship of energy to the spiritual state of the individual, as well as the physical state. I would learn a lot of that by challenges I would face that would test my faith, and clarify what my belief systems were. This trip began the cracking of my spirit, to get to the meat of my heart and show me how to live and love, and to bring that joy to all that I do. I am truly grateful for that experience.

In the years to come, I would learn the importance of meditation, prayer, healthy food, natural supplements, and hormonal balance to a person's well being, trying them all on myself first. I was humbled by the inadequacies of western medicine, and marveled at nature's ability to solve most modern ailments, but then again, the root cause was what one brought upon one's self, as we are vibrational beings that will call to ourselves that which our spirit truly desires, even if that desire is death.

While western medicine has a basic arsenal of typically chemical medicines, and surgical options, too often the human element is left out, thankfully this is beginning to change. Due to the constraints of the modern physician on time and reimbursement, many

Mystic Awakening of an American Physician
Linda Hostalek, D.O.

patients don't feel their needs met and will continue to loop until they find the relationship to the mind, body and spirit. We are energetic, vibrational beings. Our energy field should resonate with the natural world's vibration. Our spirit resides in our human suit, so it is important to take care of that suit. That is accomplished by making sure we take the time to rest, eat properly, drink clean pure energized water, do work that makes us fulfilled, have rewarding personal relationships, and a loving relationship with Spirit. We are more than just our body, we are more than just our mind, and as we realize that we are all connected, to each other, to the earth, to the collective consciousness of divine realization, we will realize that our actions affect all things. That is one of the reasons that both cranial osteopathy and shamanism appeal to me, they both address imbalances of the spirit, which lead to healing of the physical body.

As we rape and kill the rainforest, we do that to ourselves; when we are kind and give our love to a tree, flower or bird, we also are doing that to ourself, for every act is truly a mirror of our soul. Mother Earth is beginning to establish her supremacy and balance herself, with earthquakes, floods, droughts, fires, hurricanes, etc. When will we learn to live in balance with the earth, and love her and all her creatures? When will we truly love ourself? When we learn to give of ourselves without expecting anything in return, but instead doing the right thing because it feels right, the blessings abound.

When one lives in balance with the nature and the spirit inside, one learns to be in a more harmonious place. As you change one small thing to help your health, such as drinking pure, clean water, and you love that clean pure water, you vibrate higher, and the water vibrates higher, because the highest vibration is love. Love is the healing vibration. Love is what drives the plants to flower, the birds to sing, and our hearts to be supremely happy.

The paradigm shift is upon us. There is always more healing to do, and always more love to fill our hearts. My prayer is that this shift will change medicine to what it was in the ancient days, a mixture of science and spirit, of obtaining balance and purity, to be of

Mystic Awakening of an AmericanPhysician
Linda Hostalek, D.O.

useful service to humanity, as well as to one's self and family.

When we are happy we are in a healthy vibration. And healing does not always mean 'cure'. As we realize that we are more than our body, and explore our relationship with all that is, and come to a peace in our spirit, we can heal. We can heal our self, our family, our world. There may still be problems, but together we truly can overcome everything, one vibration at a time.

We live in a time where we have many uncertainties. When your spirit is strong, you can see the changes as a new beginning. And in love, trust, and appreciation for all that is, adopt a new way of life, to be a part of the solution in your own way, and your heart will show you how as we enter this new pacha, or time cycle that has been prophesied through many traditions all over the globe.

The time when we meet ourselves is our next becoming. That is happening now, and the minerals, animals and plants are teaching us, if we only have the ears to hear. Spirit is talking to us from the other side, through the veil which is getting thinner each day. The goal of a good medicine person is to walk in both sides simultaneously.

The last gift Richard gave me was an introduction to the other side via the sacred plant medicines. The veil was lifted and I was shown how humans are light beings and when we are in 'dis-ease', those light cords get tangled, and that the job of a healer is to untangle those light cords and make them smooth and healthy again. The experiences of connective-ness to all that is rocked my world and changed me forever. I needed some time to let these experiences sink into my everyday life. As I was shown the patterns of everything from the sacred geometry in a nautilus shell to the solar system, the knowingness that is an integral part of all, the mystic awakens. This experience prepared me for what was to come next, and my gratitude continues to this day......

Mystic Awakening of an AmericanPhysician
Linda Hostalek, D.O.

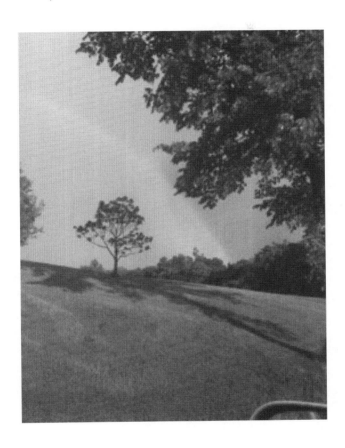

Mystic Awakening of an AmericanPhysician

Epilogue

Thank you Pachamama, Mother Earth and Great
Spirit, Great Creator, God, for the lessons I've been
taught. Thank you to Richard, and to Jose Luis, my
mentor and dear friend who taught me more than I
could ever write down. Thank you to the plant
medicines, who will be the subject of the next book,
for teaching me the multidimensionality of this reality.
I am grateful to all my teachers, both in western
medicine, especially those who taught me cranial, and
to those who taught me in the mystery schools, who
taught me to weave the sacred into the profane. To
the rock people, whose vibration echoes the
beginning of time and is the keeper of the records,
and to the animals, who know how to live in the kay-

pacha, this reality, while keeping their anima, their spirit, intact. And much appreciation and love to the plant kingdom, for its healing vibrations via it's many foods and medicines, teaching us humans about abundance, healing and love.

It is through the eyes of spirit that we can see the divine in everything, I pray we can all open our eyes, and see that we are so loved and that we create everything, including the destructive things of this world. That means we can change it back to a place of love, light and harmony, if we align our spirits with this vibration.

Buckminster Fuller said his life was an experiment, to see what one man could do. Perhaps we could all live our life as an experiment, to boldly love this 'spaceship earth,' and to care for the creatures, large and small, that make up this environment. We truly are the oceans, the mountains, the jungles, deserts, and plains. We are the babbling mountain brooks, the glaciers, and the stars. It is time to reclaim out spiritual selves, and that of the world. Please join me in living your life in line with Spirit, to the best of your ability. Marvel at the beauty of a tree, the sunset, or the ocean. Know that that Spirit that lives there, lives in you too. Honor that Spirit, honor your self, honor all life, and come to know that you are here for a special purpose, unique to you.

Mystic Awakening of an AmericanPhysician